THE NEW INTERNATIONAL

WEBSTER'S POCKET MEDICAL & FIRST AID DICTIONARY

OF THE ENGLISH LANGUAGE

■■■■■ ◆◆◆ ■■■■■

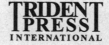

TRIDENT PRESS INTERNATIONAL

Published by

Trident Press International

1998 EDITION

Cover Design Copyright © Trident Press International
Text Copyright © 1997 J. Radcliffe

ISBN 1-888-777-22-2 Deluxe Edition
ISBN1-888-777-32-X Hardcover Edition
ISBN1-888-777-40-0 Paperback Edition

abacterial
Descriptive of that which is not caused or typified by the presence of bacteria.

abdomen, abdominal cavity
That part of the human body comprising the lower portion of the ***trunk***, defined by the lower section of the backbone and the muscles of the back, and abdominal muscles at the sides and front. The ***diaphragm*** forms the top of the cavity and the pelvic basin forms the bottom.

The abdominal cavity contains several important organs: the ***liver*** in the upper right portion; the ***stomach*** and the ***spleen*** in the upper left portion; the small and large ***intestines*** in the lower portion; the ***kidneys***, one on each side in the back; and the ***urinary bladder*** in the pelvic region. There are also major blood vessels and other smaller organs in the abdominal cavity.

abduct
To move away from the midline of the body.

abduction
Descriptive of the movement of a limb or part of a limb away from the midline of the body, as, for example, when the arm is lifted away from the side of the body. Similarly, separation of the fingers or toes is called abduction.

See also, ***adduction.***

abductor
A muscle that controls movement away from the midline of the body

aberrant
Deviating from the usual or normal, as behavior of a

1

mental patient.

aberration

Something *abnormal*, as of the functioning of the mind or a physical disorder.

abeyance

A lessening, as of a symptom, usually temporary.

ablation

Separation or removal of a part of the body by surgery.

ablution

Washing of the body.

abortion

The untimely termination of a pregnancy, either by natural or artificial means.

abnormal

Descriptive of that which is unusual; not conforming to the normal.

abrade

To wear down by rubbing, as the skin.

abrasion

An injury caused by rubbing the surface of the skin.

abscess

A swollen, inflamed area of body tissue, often tender or painful, in which pus has gathered.

The abscess is the result of the body's natural response to bacterial infection or an irritant, such as a splinter.

Leukocytes, or white blood cells gather in the area to fight the infection: as the dead bacteria, dead leukocytes, etc. build up to form *pus*, they create pressure and discomfort results. Pressing along the line of least resistance, the abscess pushes toward the

2

surface. Eventually the abscess will burst of its own accord, but may be lanced by a doctor. It is inadvisable to attempt to puncture the abscess before it is ready, as such action may spread the infection.

absorption

The process of assimilating food or other substances into the body. Absorption may take place by a number of means, as through the gastro-intestinal tract, through the skin, or through the mucous membranes of the eyes, nose, etc.

Food and drink taken by mouth pass through the esophagus to the stomach, and finally to the small intestine where the bulk of absorption of food takes place.

Many drugs are absorbed in the same way: taken by mouth, they are carried to the small intestine where they pass through the intestinal wall and enter the bloodstream.

Drugs can be absorbed through the skin and the mucous membranes.

Light rays are absorbed by the body through the skin.

abstinence

Voluntarily doing without or denying oneself of an indulgence such as of certain food or drink.

abuse

Immoderate or inappropriate use of something, as of a drug.

acapnia

A lack of carbon dioxide in the blood or tissues of the body.

accelerator
An agent that speeds the action of, as a medication.
A nerve or muscle that intensifies a body function.

acclimate
To adjust to new conditions, such as temperature or environment.

accommodation
The adjustment of the lens of the eyes to adapt to available light so as to see clearly in bright or sub-dued light, and to distinguish objects that are near and those that are far away.

When looking at a close object, the lens of the eye thickens and becomes more convex in order to focus the light from that object on the *retina*; for a distant object, the lens contracts to bring the light from the object into focus.

Over the years, the lens may lose some of its elasticity, limiting the ability to focus, often evidenced by the tendency to hold reading matter further away or the need to wear glasses for reading.

accouchement
Confinement during childbirth.

accretion
The process of growth.

ache
A continuous or steady dull pain.

Achilles tendon
The tendon that attaches the bone of the heel to the muscles of the calf of the leg.

acne
An inflammation of the sebaceous glands, or oil-secreting organs, of the skin, manifested by

eruptions of hard, inflamed pimples. The condition is most common among teenagers. The oil, sebum, is a fatty substance that normally helps maintain the texture of the skin.

Increased production of androgens, or male sex hormones, in both males and females during puberty causes the sebaceous glands to become especially active and secrete large amounts of sebum that is unusually thick. This sebum has a tendency to block the glands and hair follicles. When this occurs, the follicles become clogged with sebum and cellular debris.

Usually the condition is only alleviated by time, fading as the individual reaches adulthood.

Washing gently with a mild soap and water often helps by removing some of the bacteria and debris. Medication is sometimes effective for reducing symptoms, as is exposure to sunlight that tends to dry up the eruptions.

acoustic nerve

The nerve that serves to transmit images related to hearing and balance from the inner ear to the brain.

acquired

Descriptive of that which is developed or modified by environmental influence, in contrast to that which is inherited.

acrid

Of a taste or odor that is sharp and unpleasant.

acquired immune deficiency syndrome See *AIDS*

acrophobia

An excessive dread of high places. Some fear of heights is natural as part of the human defense

mechanism in consideration of the possible consequences of falling. Acrophobia, however, is an un-
reasonable magnification of this normal fear, as the
acrophobic may be terrified even in a high place
where the possibility of falling is nil. Acrophobia can
be disabling when it precludes work or social functions that involve going above the ground floor of a
building.

ACTH
AdrenoCorticoTropic Hormone; an essential hormone
produced by the pituitary gland, that lies at the base
of the brain. ACTH provides the link between the
pituitary gland and the cortex, or covering, of the
adrenal glands that secretes vital hormones essential for maintaining the body's biochemical balance.
See also, *endocrinology*.

acuity
Keen insight or perception.

acupressure
A technique for applying pressure to various points
on the body in order to alleviate pain or deal with
disease.

acupuncture
The ancient technique of inserting the tips of long
needles into the skin and manipulating them to relieve pain or treat disease.

acute
Sudden or severe, although of short duration, as
contrasted to *chronic.*

acute bronchitis
A respiratory tract infection that causes inflammation of the trachea and the bronchi.

Beginning with a dry cough that turns to one producing mucus, the infection may cause discomfort during inhalation. Treatment generally is the same as for coughs or colds—cough suppressants and plenty of liquids. Moistening the air with a humidifier will help clear passages of mucus. A physician should be consulted if symptoms persist or if there is a possibility of more serious infection.

adaptation
The process of adjusting to conditions, as by an organism.

addiction
Dependence or compulsive use on a habit–forming or harmful substance.

addictive
Descriptive of a substance that is inherently habit–forming.

Addison's disease
A condition that occurs when the adrenal glands cease to function properly and fail to produce adequate quantities of the hormones called steroids.
The symptoms of Addison's disease are weakness, fatigue, and increased pigmentation of the skin. Further symptoms may include weight loss, dehydration, low blood pressure, and nausea.

adduction
Descriptive of the movement of a limb or part of a limb toward the midline of the body, as, for example, when an outstretched arm is brought back to the side of the body. Similarly, bringing a separated finger or toe back to its normal position is called adduction.

The muscles involved in such movement are referred to as *adductors*. See also, ***abduction***.

adenitis

Inflammation of a lymph gland or node. The lymph glands are scattered throughout the body, mainly concentrated at the side of the neck, in the armpits and in the groin, to aid the body in defending against infection.

adenocarcinoma

A common form of cancerous tumor, originating in glandular tissue, mainly in the stomach, large intestine, gallbladder, pancreas, uterus or the prostate gland. The tumor may also start in the breast or in the lungs.

If not detected and treated promptly, adenocarcinomas commonly spread to other parts of the body via the blood or lymphatic systems The secondary tumor formed by such spreading to another site has the same appearance as that of the original tumor, aiding in further diagnosis if the location of the original tumor is unknown.

adenoids

A mass of lymphoid tissue located at the entrance to the throat, above the tonsils. The adenoids contain specialized white blood cells that help provide protection against diseases of the respiratory system.

The adenoids may become enlarged by throat infections as the tonsils do, and sometimes, as a result of repeated infections or allergies, they remain enlarged, obstructing the nasal passage. There is some reluctance to remove them by surgery, however, because of the protective nature of their function and the fact that they begin to shrink away at an early age, so that they are usually gone during adolescence.

adenoma

A benign, or non–malignant tumor originating in glandular tissue, as contrasted to *adenocarcinoma*. An adenoma is usually harmless, although it may cause discomfort or pain. It remains isolated and will not spread or destroy other tissue.

adenosis

Disease of a gland, particularly the abnormal development of glandular tissue.

adhesion

The joining of tissue that is ordinarily separate.

Tissue that joins other, normally separated, tissue.

adipose tissue

Fatty tissue that occurs throughout the body, mainly directly under the skin, acting as an insulation and a source of energy. It is thickest in those parts of the body most liable to sudden trauma, such as the buttocks and feet where it acts as a shock absorber.

Adipose tissue in bone marrow supports the arteries and veins; in the joints and muscles, it deters injury from sudden shock; it provides cushion and support for the heart and lungs; keeps the intestines warm; and protects the kidneys from shock.

An excess of adipose tissue can be dangerous, particularly around the heart or lungs where it adds weight to the organ and restricts its movement.

adjuvant

A substance added to a medication or serum to

intensify or aid its action.

adrenal gland
One of the two glands that each lie above a kidney
and secrete hormones to control certain functions of
the body.

Hormones from the adrenal glands assist in the
maintenance of the body's fluid balance, enhance
the body's ability to cope with stress, and are vital to
the body's metabolism and sexual development.

adrenalectomy
Excision of one or both of the adrenal glands by surgery.

adult
One who is fully developed or mature, especially
physically and intellectually.

aerobe
A microorganism that requires oxygen to sustain life.

aerobic
Occurring only in the presence of oxygen, as an organism that requires oxygen to survive.

Involving the consumption or use of oxygen such as
aerobic exercise.

aerobics, aerobic exercise
Exercise designed to condition the body by stimulating oxygen consumption in the muscles and thereby
making them work more efficiently.

The exercises themselves range from mild exertion
such as by brisk walking to more strenuous activities such as jogging or jumping rope. The main requirement for successful conditioning is that the activity be carried on long enough to increase the heart
rate somewhat.

As with all exercise plans it is wise to start slowly and gradually increase intensity. Anyone who has not exercised for a long time or with a condition that may be worsened by improper exercise should first consult a physician.

afebrile
Of a condition that is not characterized or distinguished by fever.

aftercare
Care or treatment of one who is convalescing from an illness, operation, etc.

agoraphobia
An irrational dread of open or public places; a fear of leaving a place considered safe, as the home, manifested by a feeling of panic, often accompanied by a rapid heartbeat, sweating and trembling.

ague
A bout of chills and fever alternating at somewhat regular intervals.

AIDS
Acquired Immune Deficiency Syndrome, a disease that attacks the body's immune system, rendering it unable to fight disease.

AIDS is caused by a microorganism called the human immunodeficiency virus (HIV), transmitted in body fluids through sexual intercourse, the use of non sterile hypodermic needles, and contact with infected blood. A pregnant woman also may transmit the disease to the fetus.

Early symptoms include low grade fever, swollen lymph nodes, fatigue, weight loss, and diarrhea. The AIDS victim suffers from an impaired immune system, and thus is susceptible to many diseases, including various cancers, skin infections, and fungal infections. Many of the victims develop a cancer known as Kaposi's sarcoma, which often appears as purplish bumps on the skin.

Some individuals may unknowingly be carriers without exhibiting any symptoms of the disease. Blood tests can indicate exposure to the disease, although not all individuals with positive test results will contract AIDS.

It is possible to limit the potential for exposure to the virus, as by restricting the number of one's sexual partners, using condoms, and avoiding contact with hypodermic needles or blood that may be contaminated. It is common practice to give blood in advance of elective surgery, so that any transfusions will be of one's own blood although thorough testing has virtually eliminated contamination in the blood supply. There is no evidence to indicate that the virus is transmitted through casual contacts.

albinism

A condition characterized by a lack of natural pigment in the skin, causing an unnaturally pale appearance. The victim has a low tolerance for exposure to the sun and may exhibit an excessive sensitivity to bright light.

albumen

The white of an egg.
Albumin.

albumin

One of the two major proteins of the blood, formed in the liver from ingested food.

Albumin is water–soluble and found in various forms in animals, egg white and vegetables. See also, *globulin.*

albuminuria

The presence of **albumin** in the urine, often a sign of kidney malfunction. **Proteinuria** is virtually the same as albuminuria, since albumin is the only protein detected in significant amounts in the urine.

alcohol

Alcohol refers to any of a class of organic compounds containing one or more hydroxyl groups, as *ethyl alcohol*, obtained by the fermentation of sugar, used in medicine and beverages, or *methyl alcohol*, synthesized from carbon monoxide and hydrogen, used as a fuel, solvent, etc.; a colorless, volatile liquid.

alcoholism

A disease caused by the excess consumption of alcoholic beverages.

Small doses of alcohol cause a feeling of relaxation, some loss of inhibitions and stimulation of the appetite due to an increase in the flow of gastric juices. Larger doses can impair speech and muscular coordination, and may irritate the stomach lining. A very large amount can produce severe depression of the central nervous system and may be fatal.

Regular ingestion of large quantities of alcohol can create a dependency and have injurious effects on the organs of the body, especially of the liver.

algesia

Sensitivity to pain.

alimentary

Relating to nourishment or nutrition, or to the

alkalosis

body's system for the intake of food, digestion, and the removal of waste.

alkalosis

An excessive concentration of alkali, or bicarbonate, in the body fluids.

Metabolic alkalosis normally is the result of the loss of hydrochloric acid from the stomach caused by protracted vomiting or taking an excessive amount of antacids for an upset stomach. Usually, the condition is alleviated when the kidneys have enough fluid to adjust the amount of alkali in the blood.

Respiratory alkalosis is caused by excessive exhalation of carbon dioxide, usually caused by hysterical over breathing that can often be corrected by breathing into a paper bag so that carbon dioxide breathed out is breathed in again.

Alkalosis may be characterized by dizziness and jerky muscular contractions.

allergen

Any substance that causes an allergic response in the body's immune system.

allergist

One who specializes in the causes and symptoms of allergy and treatment for them.

allergy

Excessive sensitivity to a substance, as pollen, feathers, or dust, or a chemical, such as a detergent, cosmetic or drug.

Allergy is the cause of hay fever and hives, and may be the cause of many cases of asthma, eczema and sinusitis.

Allergic reactions are an exaggeration of the normal

immune response to bacteria, virus, etc. Normally, the body responds to invasion by forming antibodies to fight the invader. The allergic response is similar, except that the antibodies react with the allergen, or invader substance, to cause the body to release chemicals that create undesirable side affects. Allergic reactions are most common in the respiratory tract and the skin, though they may also affect the digestive system.

allergy and immunology

The study of the diagnosis and treatment of disorders that relate to the body's ability to resist threatening substances.

Immunologists, for example, may search for ways to prevent cancer by modifying the immune system to reject cancerous growth or to bring about selective operation of the immune system so that the body will accept an organ transplant.

Immunologists who deal with allergies are concerned with identifying environmental irritants that cause symptoms, and devising treatment. Allergies may be alleviated by a change of environment to eliminate the irritant, the use of drugs to relieve symptoms, or a program of desensitization that involves the injection of minute amounts of the irritant to make the immune system less sensitive to it.

alleviative

Of that which eases the discomfort of illness or disease, as contrasted to a *curative*.

aloe

A plant of the lily family that is prized for its curative powers.

alogia
An inability to speak, especially when attributed to brain damage.

alviolitis
Infection of the alveoli of the lungs.

alvioli (singular, **alviolus**)
Small cavities in the body such as the air cells of the lungs.

Alzheimer's disease
A disease caused by presenile brain atrophy. Atrophy, or shrinking, of the brain may be expected in old age; *presenile brain atrophy* is the premature shrinking of the brain that causes slowing of the mental processes, beginning with forgetfulness and progressing to irrationality.

The first symptoms are small memory lapses, usually involving lack of recall for recent events. As they grow more serious, a person may forget the name of a close relative or friend, get lost traveling between familiar places, misplace articles, recheck tasks that has been done, or repeatedly ask questions that have already been answered.

As the disease grows worse, Alzheimer victim becomes confused, frustrated, and irritable. Endless repetition of unnecessary actions is also characteristic of the disease. Some victims may become extremely agitated with little or no provocation.

amalgam
An alloy of mercury used in cementing fillings for the teeth.

ambidextrous
Being equally proficient with the use of either hand.

amblyopia

Defective eyesight without any apparent defect of the eye. The condition may be temporary or permanent and it may be partial or result in total blindness in the affected eye.

Amblyopia may be caused by poisons in the system, as from alcohol, tobacco, lead, arsenic compounds, petroleum derivatives, etc. Strokes often cause some loss of vision when there is damage to the portion of the brain that controls eyesight.

amenorrhea

A lack of menstruation. *Primary amenorrhea* refers to a condition in which menstruation has never occurred. *Secondary amenorrhea* refers to a cessation of menstruation in a woman who has previously been menstruating.

Secondary amenorrhea is probably most commonly caused by pregnancy and lactation. It may also be due to anemia brought on by heavy menstrual blood loss in the past, ovarian failure, certain pituitary diseases, an emotional disturbance or even a distinctive change in life style.

amentia

Mental retardation; a congenital mental deficiency. See also, *dementia*.

amino acid

Any of the group of organic compounds that form the basic constituents of protein.

aminoacidemia

A condition characterized by an increase in the concentration of amino acids in the blood.

aminoaciduria
A condition characterized by an increase in the concentration of amino acids in the urine.
amnesia
A loss of memory that may be temporary or permanent, caused by damage to the brain or psychological reaction.

An injury to the head that involves loss of consciousness may result in some loss of memory. Often the memories of a period before and after the injury are blanked out. The memory may return as the victim recovers from the injury, but parts of memory may never be recovered. Similar loss of memory can occur in the case of severe **trauma**, or injury, that does not involve the head.

Abrupt memory loss without injury or illness is usually the result of a psychological disorder; a person wandering aimlessly with no recollection of name or address is probably suffering from *hysterical amnesia* brought on by emotional stress.

Disease or injury can affect short–term or long–term memory, or both.

Memory for most of one's life is normally continuous, although there is usually little or no recollection of infancy. In old age, the memory of recent events may be faulty, while memories from the distant past remain intact.

Short–term memory loss is also a symptom of chronic alcoholism and some brain diseases such as Alzheimer's.
amniocentesis
Drawing off a sample of the amniotic fluid from the

womb of a pregnant woman in order to examine it. The amniotic fluid is the medium in which the fetus lies and contains some cells from the fetus that can be analyzed to detect a number of abnormalities.

amputation

The cutting off of a part of the body, usually a limb or part of a limb.

Amputation may be caused by accident, as in an automobile or industrial plant, or it may be part of a surgical procedure necessitated by injury or disease.

anabolism

The conversion of food into living tissue by the body; part of the total metabolic process. See also, *catabolism*.

anaerobic

Of that which occurs or exists without oxygen.

analgesia

Relief from pain without loss of consciousness.

Analgesics, or drugs that produce analgesia, are of three types: those that act directly on the source of the pain, those that act on the brain, and those that are specific, that is, they act on a particular illness or disease.

The most common analgesics are those in the first group, such as acetaminophen or aspirin, used to combat relatively mild pain. In addition to its analgesic action, aspirin is known for its ability to reduce fever and inflammation; for some, however, it may cause an upset stomach or some other reaction. Acetaminophen is milder, but is not as effective for reducing fever or inflammation.

The second group, far more potent and with a

19

potential for abuse and addiction, are dispensed only by prescription. They include substances such as morphine, methadone and codeine.

The analgesics in the third group, as noted above, act on specifics, such as a migraine or a certain types of neuralgia.

Analgesia can also be uncontrolled, as from a disease of the sensory system or from an overdose of alcohol.

anaphylactic shock
A severe reaction of the body to certain vaccines, antibiotics, insect stings or other antigens that may cause a state of total collapse.

Normally the body reacts to the presence of an ***antigen***, or foreign substance, by creating an ***antibody***, or compound, that can render the foreign substance harmless. In some persons, sensitivity to certain antigens triggers a reaction that is harmful and can be dangerous. Such sensitivity is cumulative, in that subsequent attacks are worse than the previous attack.

Anaphylactic shock is most readily evidenced by difficulty in breathing, and failure to act quickly may prove fatal—the victim requires immediate medical attention.

Any significant reaction to a shot or an insect bite should be quickly brought to the attention of a physician.

anatomy
A study of the structure of organisms.

ancillary
Of a substance or procedure that is supplemental.

androgen

A substance that promotes the development of secondary male characteristics

anemia

A shortage of red blood cells or a deficiency in hemoglobin, the pigment in red blood cells that carries oxygen.

The symptoms of anemia are not distinctive, and the condition may not be detected unless it is severe. The sufferer may experience fatigue, shortness of breath, rapid heart rate, headaches, loss of appetite, dizziness, and weakness. Very severe cases of anemia may exhibit swollen ankles, a rapid weak pulse and pale clammy skin.

Anemia can be caused by inadequate materials for the manufacture of red blood cells, the inability of bone marrow to manufacture the cells, excessive or untimely destruction of the cells, or inherited abnormalities.

A lack of raw materials, such as iron, vitamin B_{12}, or folic acid can inhibit the production of hemoglobin. Iron, for example, may be lost in excessive bleeding, or be unavailable in a diet lacking in dark green vegetables, egg yolk, meat, seafood, or dried beans. Illness or disease may render the body unable to absorb the vital materials even though they are present.

The function of the bone marrow may be inhibited by disease, exposure to radioactivity, or drugs.

Red blood cells may be destroyed by excessive bleeding, disease, infection, or a mismatched blood transfusion.

anesthesia

In inherited, or congenital conditions, there is an abnormality in the red blood cell that inhibits effective function, such as sickle cell anemia, in which the blood cells cannot carry sufficient oxygen to the body and are inclined to break down easily.

Conditions such as bleeding ulcers, cancer, and alcoholism are likely to cause one or more types of anemia.

anesthesia

A diminished or lost sense of feeling, especially the sensations of pain and touch. Anesthesia can be brought on by disease, trauma, damage to the nervous system, or the action of drugs.

Anesthesia usually refers to the administering of a drug to produce a reduced state of sensitivity in order to perform a surgical operation, or to the drug so administered.

anesthesiology

The science of the administration of drugs to reduce or limit sensitivity. The anesthesiologist specializes in administering those drugs that limit sensation, or the body's ability to sense pain.

aneurysm

A bulge, or swelling, in an artery that has been weakened by disease or injury.

The primary danger associated with an aneurysm is that of rupture of the blood vessel, causing internal bleeding that can prove fatal.

Aneurysms occur most often in: the aorta, the largest artery in the body; the artery behind the knee; and the arteries at the base of the brain. The aneurysm may be detected in the abdomen as a pulsating mass that is very tender, and at the back of the knee, one that is painful. In a neck artery, there may be interference with nerves serving the eye, causing double vision, as well as a pulsating sound that the victim may detect.

A dissecting aneurysm is one in which the blood runs between the walls of the artery, sometimes eventually reentering the main vessel. A dissecting aneurysm in the chest will cause severe pain in the area and often symptoms resembling a heart attack. In the abdomen, pain may be severe in the area and radiate to the back, accompanied by a loss of blood to the legs.

angina pectoris

A dull pressure or pain in the center of the chest that may be accompanied by a burning sensation not unlike indigestion and may radiate down the left arm; an indication that the heart muscle is not getting enough oxygen during a period of stress or exertion

The pain of an attack of angina pectoris is usually not as severe as that of a heart attack, and the heart muscles are not damaged. The pain will usually recede quickly if the victim stops all activity and rests. Although an attack of angina is not a heart attack, the experience indicates that the individual may be a likely candidate for heart attack.

A number of conditions can prevent the heart muscle from getting enough blood to supply adequate oxygen. The most common condition is narrowing of the coronary artery due to *atherosclerosis*. Physical or mental stress can hasten onset of the condition.

Whatever the suspected cause, a physician should be consulted.

Angina is usually treated by altering lifestyle to reduce stress and strain on the heart. Smoking, overeating and overexertion should be avoided. Regular exercise is necessary, but it should be tailored to the condition, avoiding those activities that place sudden, severe demands on the heart.

angiocardiography

An x ray examination of the heart and its blood vessels that have been injected with a substance that is opaque to x rays in order to make them visible on the x–ray plate or viewing screen. This technique is also used in the diagnosis of tumors, especially of the brain.

angiography

An x ray examination of blood vessels that have been injected with a substance that is opaque to x rays.

angioma

A tumor made up of mostly blood and lymph vessels.

angioplasty

Any of a number of surgical techniques for the repairing of damaged blood vessels.

ankylosis

A condition characterized by stiffness or immobility of a joint caused by fusion of its parts as a consequence of injury or surgery.

anorexia nervosa

Anorexia is a lack of appetite, or desire for food; *anorexia nervosa* is an *aversion* to food.

The condition usually begins as an attempt to lose weight, but is then carried to extremes. The subject continues to lose weight, and may suffer from severe vitamin and mineral deficiency. The condition is often worsened by vomiting, the use of purgatives and excessive exercise. If allowed to continue the victim will literally starve to death, while convinced that his or her diet is adequate.

antacid
A medication that neutralizes acidity.

anthrax
An infectious disease that commonly infects cattle, goats or sheep and can be transmitted to man. Humans contract the infection from the spores that survive in contaminated wool, hair or hides. Hygienic methods of handling these raw materials have diminished the spread of the disease.
Infection can affect the skin, where it is characterized by itching pustules that turn black as the infection spreads. The infection also has a tendency to attack the lungs.

antibiotic
A medication designed to destroy or restrain the growth of an organism.
That with tends to hinder or destroy life.

antibody
A chemical compound produced by the body to combine with and neutralize a particular foreign substance, called an *antigen*, entering the body.
The antibody created in reaction to a particular antigen is a unique one, effective only in defense against that antigen. Its purpose is to overcome an attack of infectious matter and to stand ready to ward off future attacks.

anticoagulant

The first time a particular bacteria invades, the body formulates an antibody. By the time the infection has run its course, there are often enough of the specific antibodies remaining in the blood to ward off the second attack, perhaps for life. Such is the basis for immunization, that which introduces dead or weakened bacteria into the body so that it will develop the necessary antibodies while experiencing few or none of the symptoms of the disease.

anticoagulant
A medication that slows clotting or coagulation of the blood.

antidote
A substance that counteracts the effects of a poison.

antifungal
A substance that checks the growth of a fungal infection.

antigen
Any substance the immune system identifies as a potential threat that starts the reaction leading to the production of a special *antibody*.
Antigens are contained in bacteria and viruses, blood from an incompatible blood group, and sera injected into the body for the treatment or prevention of infectious diseases.

antihistamine
Any medication that arrests the action of a histamine, such as those used in treating a cold or hay fever.

antipyretic
Any medication that tends to reduce fever, such as aspirin.

antiseptic
Any substance that inhibits the action of bacteria.
antitoxin
A substance that neutralizes a specific toxin that is released by bacteria.
anuria
Lack of urination caused by kidney failure or by a blockage.
anxiety
Fear or apprehension about some future possibility. Anxiety is a normal response to anything that is of concern, the outcome of which is uncertain, as a first day of school or a trip to the dentist. It may, however, become excessive and irrational. Concern about making a good impression when meeting people, for example, is a form of anxiety; such anxiety is unhealthy, however, when apprehension is so great that one refuses to meet new people. Excessive anxiety about pollution, auto accidents, etc. can trap one in the home without hope of reprieve.
aorta
The main artery of the body, that extends from the left ventricle of the heart to begin the distribution of blood throughout the rest of the body.
aphagia
A lack of ability to swallow.
aphasia
Partial or total loss of the ability to speak coherently, especially to connect words and ideas, caused by stroke or other illness.
aphrasia
Loss of the ability to form words in a sentences or in

aplasia

a comprehensible pattern.

aplasia

The defective or incomplete formation of an organ.

apnea

A temporary stopping of breathing.

apoplexy See *stroke*.

apothecary

A pharmacist. An outdated term that is now used mainly to describe the system of standards used to calibrate preparations made by the pharmacist, as an *apothecary's weight* or *apothecary's measure*.

appendage

An accessory or additional part; an outgrowth.

appendectomy

The surgical excision of the appendix.

appendicitis

Inflammation of the appendix, a small growth at the end of the large intestine, near its juncture with the small intestine.

The appendix serves no apparent purpose and the operation is quite simple. An infected appendix, however, can burst, with serious consequences.

Appendicitis usually produces a dull or sharp pain in the abdomen that may be intensified by coughing, sneezing, or even moving. This is usually accompanied by a feeling of nausea and constipation, although diarrhea is not infrequent. As the pain becomes constant, it may move to the lower right side of the abdomen over the appendix or even to the back. The area around the appendix may become very tender. At this stage the appendix is likely to become so swollen that it bursts, infecting the surrounding organs and creating a potentially life threatening situation.

Symptoms vary from person to person, as does the location of the appendix. When there is severe abdominal pain that persists, consult a physician as quickly as possible.

appliance
A device that is attached to the body for some purpose, as one designed to replace a missing limb.

apyretic
Lacking indications of fever; *afebrile*.

aqueous
Containing or resembling water.

arbovirus
Any of a number of viruses that are transmitted by insects.

arrhythmia
An irregular heartbeat.

arteriole
Any of the small endings of an artery that connect to capillaries. See *blood vessels*.

arteriosclerosis
Any condition in which the walls of the arteries are thickened and made rigid, making them unable to process an adequate supply of blood. Commonly called *hardening of the arteries*. See also, *atherosclerosis*.

artery
Any of the vessels that deliver blood from the heart throughout the body. See also, *blood vessels*.

arthralgia
Pain in a joint.

arthrectomy
Surgical removal or replacement of a joint.
arthritis
Any inflammation of the *joints*.
Arthritis causes swelling, pain, and stiffness in the joints. Damp weather, emotional stress excess weight, and abuse of the joints at work or play can make symptoms more pronounced.
The onset of arthritis is brought about by damage to the smooth surfaces where two bones join caused by injury, a progressive wearing away with age, or illness, such as crystal deposits from gout or tumors that push the joint out of position. The most common cause is *rheumatoid arthritis* which causes inflammation in the synovium, a thin membrane that lines and lubricates the joint. The inflammation ultimately destroys the elastic tissue that lines the joint, the cartilage. The cartilage is replaced by scar tissue, and the joint becomes swollen, deformed and painful.
The most effective treatment for arthritis includes drug therapy, exercise, and rest. Aspirin is the drug most commonly prescribed for arthritis—two or three tablets several times a day may reduce inflammation and relieve pain. Non aspirin pain relievers may also be effective. Daily exercise is important to preserve mobility in the arthritic joints. Moist heat is often recommended to reduce pain and improve mobility.
arthrology
The branch of medical science that deals with the structure and ailments of joints.

arthroplasty
The surgical repair or replacement of a joint.
In some cases where joints have become stiff and painful as the result of disease or injury, the joint may be excised by cutting away the damaged portions of bone. Such surgery leaves scar tissue to fill the gap and although the pain is relieved, the joint may be unstable.
In other cases, it is possible to replace the joint or a portion of the joint that has been excised. Replacement surgery has been particularly successful in the replacement of the hip joint.

articulate
To speak distinctly or having the ability to speak distinctly.
To connect or be connected by a joint.

articulation
Clear speech.
The manner in which parts are connected by a joint.

artificial insemination
An attempt to induce pregnancy without sexual contact. Semen is collected from the male and deposited in the cervix or uterus of the female at the time of ovulation.

asbestosis
An inflammation of the lungs caused by the inhalation of asbestos particles.
Certain types of the mineral *asbestos* do not burn or conduct heat or electricity, and are therefore used in the making of heat and fire resistant products, and insulation. Asbestosis is commonly contracted by those who work with asbestos or in some other way

are exposed to fine particles of asbestos in the air. The asbestos particles irritate the lungs and cause shortness of breath and coughing. The victim may also suffer loss of appetite, weight loss, and bouts of fatigue. After a time, often many years, the sufferer is likely to contract tuberculosis and cancer.

ascorbic acid See *Vitamin C*.

asepsis
The condition of being completely free of germs.

aspartame
A sugar substitute.

aspermatism, aspermia
The inability to produce semen.

asphyxia
Suffocation; a lack of oxygen in the blood caused by interference with respiration, usually involving loss of consciousness.

Drowning is probably the most common cause of asphyxia when water blocks the passage of air to the lungs. The air passage may also be shut off by accidental inhalation of food, blockage of the throat by swelling from an infection, or strangulation.

Other causes include the inhalation of air that contains too little oxygen, air containing poison gases, and electric shock.

aspirate
To draw out by the use of suction. The material drawn out.

assimilate
To take in and absorb by the system, as nourishment or a medication.

asthenia
A loss or lack of body strength or stamina.

asthma
A respiratory disorder characterized by difficulty in breathing.

Asthma attacks may be set off by an allergy, infection, overexertion, inhaling cold air, or stress. In normal breathing, air enters the lungs and is expelled through the tiny bronchioles at the end of the bronchi. The asthmatic's difficulty in breathing is caused by sensitivity of the bronchioles that brings about constriction or clogging of the tubes so that spent air cannot be properly expelled, hindering the inhalation of fresh air.

Asthma attacks are unpredictable: they may last from a few minutes to a week or more; they may occur regularly or only once in a few years; they may be mild or extremely severe.

astigmatism
A condition of the eye in which imperfect curvature of the cornea or lens prevents the image on the retina to focus clearly.

In normal vision, objects are focused sharply onto the retina. When the surfaces have an incorrect curvature, the focus is distorted and parts of the image appear blurred. Although the blurring may not be apparent, the eye may constantly readjust to correct the image, causing them to tire quickly, one of the primary symptoms of astigmatism.

astringent
A preparation that tends to draw together or shrink soft organic tissue.

asymptomatic
Lacking any indication or characteristic symptoms of disorder or disease.

ataxia
Lack of muscle coordination.

Ataxia may be congenital, that is, existing from birth, or caused by injury or disease of the central nervous system. It is characterized by irregular movements of the body that are unsteady or clumsy, as an awkward manner of walking, with feet wide apart or a lack of balance

atheroma
An abnormal deposit of fatty substance in an artery.

atherosclerosis
A condition of the arteries in which blood flow is blocked by fatty deposits.

Atherosclerosis is the most common form of *arteriosclerosis*, or hardening of the arteries, and a major contributor to heart attacks and strokes.

Formation begins when the concentration of fats that are necessary to proper function of the body and always present in the bloodstream is greatly increased and begin to form fatty streaks on the artery wall. The streaks attract nodules of cholesterol. Scar tissue forms under the nodules and attracts calcium deposits that create a hard material called plaque. The lining of plaque restricts the ability of the arteries to expand and contract properly and interferes with the flow of blood. Clots may form, further restricting the flow of blood, and in extreme cases, cutting it off entirely.

Atherosclerosis is not usually apparent until the

arteries leading to a vital organ are blocked or closed off completely. Symptoms then relate to the organ that has been cut off—stoppage of blood to the heart, for example, will trigger a heart attack; closing off arteries to the head may cause dizziness, blindness or a stroke.

Aside for treatment of the symptoms caused by atherosclerosis, and surgical procedure to bypass clogged arteries, the only treatments for the disease itself are probably of greater value in prevention, such as those of losing weight, reducing cholesterol in the diet, avoiding smoking and exercising in moderation.

athlete's foot

A fungal infection of the foot.

Athlete's foot is characterized by an itching, burning, or stinging feeling, especially between the toes where the skin often reddens and cracks. Peeling of the skin may occur, as well.

Treatment generally involves any of a number of salves, powders or liquids available from the drugstore without a prescription.

Athlete's foot can usually be prevented by eliminating the warm, moist environment in which the fungus thrives. The key is to dry feet well, especially between the toes, after taking a shower; change socks often and rotate shoes, especially in the hot, humid summer months; and use powder to keep the feet dry. Because athlete's foot is contagious, if it's not possible to avoid public showers, as in a health club, clogs should be worn in the shower and the feet dusted with an anti–fungal powder afterwards. In spite of caution, athlete's foot may easily be contracted and will often recur. If recurrence is frequent and severe, a physician should be consulted to verify that the problem is not caused by infection with similar symptoms, such as an allergic reaction to chemicals in the shoes.

atomizer
A device for spraying extremely fine particles of a liquid.

atrophy
The degeneration or wasting away of an organ or part of the body, as from disease or disuse.

attenuate
To reduce the severity of, as a disease or specific symptoms.

atypical
Not usual, as of symptoms related to a particular incidence of a disease.

audible
That can be sensed by the human ear.

audiology
The branch of medical science that deals with the hearing and the correction of hearing loss.

auditory
Of that which relates to hearing.

auscultation
Listening, as with a stethoscope to sounds within the body; sometimes, referring to the study of such sounds.

There are sounds made within the body, especially by the heart and lungs, that are characteristic of normal operation. By listening, or auscultation, the physician, with the aid of a stethoscope for amplification, is able distinguish those sounds from others that may be indicators of malfunction.

autism

A condition characterized by a preoccupation with fantasy and lack of concern for reality.

An early sign of autism is indifference to those who give care; an infant may not respond to affection or being picked up. There may be little or no interest in learning to eat, use the toilet or speak, though there is no difficulty in learning to walk.

Such children may have an excellent memory and a high level of intelligence, but no apparent concern or desire to interact with those around them. Change, such as rearranging furniture, is upsetting to them. It would appear that their perception of the everyday world is distorted and perhaps frightening, so that they seek protection in that which is familiar.

autoimmune disease

Any of a number of diseases that cause the body's immune system to produce antibodies to attack healthy tissue in the body.

autonomic

Acting involuntarily, as by control of the *autonomic nervous system* that controls bodily functions such as respiration and digestion.

autopsy

Examination of a body after death.

The autopsy, also known as a *postmortem examination* or *necropsy*, is conducted by a *pathologist* who dissects the body, usually for the purpose of determining the cause of death. Permission for the examination can be granted by a close relative, although such examination may be required in the case of death by violence or of a suspicious nature, depending on state law.

The examination is very methodical, from a thorough survey of the outer surfaces to careful examination of each organ, and includes taking samples of tissue and of the contents of the body, as urine, blood, undigested food, etc. that are kept for laboratory analysis.

AZT

AZidoThymidine; a drug used in the treatment of AIDS. Although it does not cure the disease, AZT seems to slow the growth rate of the virus.

backbone See *spinal column*.

bacteria

Any of a class of one–celled microscopic organisms, smaller than yeasts and larger than viruses, with a primitive nucleus, that multiplies by splitting in two and is able to multiply outside a living cell.

Not all bacteria are harmful and some are especially useful, as those that live in the intestines and aid in digestion, those that enrich the soil, or those used for making wine, beer, cheese, etc.

Those bacteria that produce disease are called *pathogenic*. They cause disease by invading tissue and then reproducing to destroy their surroundings, or by releasing toxins that poison the body.

Destructive bacteria are usually transmitted by direct contact, by contact with contaminated matter or by insects. Normally, the body is able to protect itself from invasion by harmful bacteria, but occasionally requires the assistance of antibiotics that destroy the organisms or prevent their multiplication.

bacteriology

The branch of medical science that deals with the forms and actions of bacteria.

balm

A soothing ointment.

barbiturate

Any of a number of compounds used as medications, especially as a sedative.

bariatrics

The study and treatment of obesity.

In addition to establishing dietary guidelines, the bariatrician is concerned with analyzing data related to the condition of being overweight or underweight in order to separate hard scientific evidence from myths about the problem.

battered-child syndrome

Physical abuse of a child by a parent, guardian, baby sitter, or anyone else in a position of trust

Abuse is often deliberate and repeated, and may be provoked by a seemingly inconsequential act.

In additional to physical injuries, the child may be deprived of food or comfort, and suffer psychological damage as a result of the abuse.

B complex See *vitamin B complex*.

bedsores

Ulcerated sores on the body of person who is bedridden for an extended period; also called *pressure sores* or *decubitus ulcers.*

When the small blood vessels that nourish the skin and underlying tissue are compressed for an extended period, they cease to function and the tissue dies. Continued pressure can cause a spread of the condition to a large area and the formation of an ulcer that may become infected.

Treatment of bedsores, like prevention, requires relief of the pressure; the patient must be allowed to recuperate on an air bed or in a net hammock.

Bell's palsy

A partial or total paralysis of one side of the face.

Bell's palsy is characterized by a lop–sided appearance to the face, mainly due to drooping of the mouth in affected side. Believed to be caused by inflammation of the nerve controlling the facial muscles, the onset of the disease is rapid. Recovery usually occurs in about a week, although it is not always complete.

bends

A painful condition in which nitrogen bubbles in the blood block the flow of blood to tissues; a symptom of decompression sickness or caisson disease.

The bends may be experienced by those moving too quickly from areas of high pressure to areas of lower pressure, as deep sea divers.

Nitrogen, present in the atmosphere, dissolves in the blood. The amount of nitrogen from the lungs that dissolves in the blood increases as pressure increases. The reverse is also true, that as the pressure decreases, the nitrogen moves from the blood to the lungs, but the process takes longer, so that if a diver surfaces too rapidly, nitrogen bubbles remain in the blood where they form air locks.

benign

Descriptive of a tumor that is not malignant, that is,

one that is expected to be of little or no harm to the body.

beriberi

A vitamin deficiency disease caused by a lack of thiamine.

Beriberi affects the circulation and the nervous system and in severe cases may cause heart failure.

bile

A yellow fluid produced by the liver to aid in the digestion, especially of fats.

Bile works in the intestine to break down fat into tiny globules that can be passed through the walls of the small intestine into the bloodstream, to provide fuel for the body.

Bile is produced continuously in the liver and stored in the gallbladder until food is ingested, at which time the bile is emptied into the intestine.

If the flow of bile is interrupted because the liver is not functioning properly or because of stoppage, digestion is impaired. Such condition can cause jaundice, a yellowing of the skin and eyes. Although jaundice is not a disease in itself it is symptomatic of a potentially severe problem and should be referred to a physician.

bilious

Of a liver disorder, especially of the excessive production of bile.

biochemistry

The study of the chemical characteristics and processes in a living organism.

biofeedback

Any technique for creating awareness of involuntary

bodily functions so as to consciously control them.

biologic, biological
Of life and the operation of living organisms.

biology
The science that deals with the study of living organisms.

biopsy
Removal of a small specimen of tissue for examination and diagnosis.

biorhythm
The regular pattern of timed sequences that alter body function such as a tendency to be more or less alert at certain times of the day or the inclination to sleep at a certain hour.

biotin See *Vitamin B complex*.

birth defect
Descriptive of an abnormality that is present at birth.

A birth defect may be *genetic*, that is, inherited from one or both parents, or it may be acquired during pregnancy or at birth.

Black Death See *bubonic plague*.

bleeder
Descriptive of a person who bleeds excessively, even from an otherwise insignificant wound.

There are some conditions, such as hemophilia, or those caused by a side affect of medication, etc. that do not allow normal clotting to occur. Persons suffering from such conditions may be in danger of bleeding to death even from the slightest of wounds. This free bleeding may be internal as well as external, a condition that warrants close observation for shock. After applying compress bandages or gauze, the person should be rushed to the nearest hospital where medical treatment can be quickly administered.

blister

A collection of fluid, as serum or blood under the outer layer of skin.

A blister may be caused by friction, as from the foot rubbing against the lining of a shoe; by heat, as from a burn; or by a caustic chemical.

An unbroken blister is little more than a petty annoyance if properly tended once the source of irritation is removed; however, a broken blister must be kept clean to prevent infection. Severe blistering should be referred to a physician for medication.

blood

A fluid that runs throughout the body by way of the arteries, veins and capillaries.

Blood is composed of serum or plasma, red cells, white cells, and platelets. Plasma is a fluid that carries the blood cells and transports nutrients to all tissues. It also transports waste products resulting from tissue activity to the organs for excretion. Red cells give color to the blood and carry oxygen. White cells aid in defending the body against infection. Platelets are essential to the formation of the blood clots necessary to stop bleeding.

A loss of blood can cause a state of physical shock that occurs because there is insufficient blood flowing through the tissues of the body to provide food and oxygen.

blood clot

blood clot
The gelatinous material formed to stem the flow of blood when a blood vessel is injured.

Normally, the lining of a blood vessel allows the blood to flow without change in its chemistry; however, when a blood vessel is ruptured and the blood comes into contact with foreign tissue, clotting begins. *Platelets* in the blood, triggered by the contact, release a chemical that begins a chain reaction involving a number of protein constituents in the blood, ending with the conversion of fibrinogen, a soluble material, to fibrin, that is insoluble. The fibrin is laid down in fine strands that collect white and red cells to form a clot.

blood vessels
Any of the passageways that carry blood: the arteries, veins and capillaries.

Oxygenated blood is carried from the heart by a large artery called the aorta. Smaller arteries branch off from this large artery, and those arteries in turn branch off into still smaller arteries. These arteries divide and subdivide until they become very small, ending in threadlike vessels known as capillaries, which extend into all the organs and tissues.

After the blood has furnished nourishment and oxygen to the tissues and organs of the body, it takes on waste products, particularly carbon dioxide. The blood returns to the heart by a system of vessels called veins. The veins connect with the arteries through the capillaries.

boil
A painful inflammation of the skin caused by a

bacterial infection; a furuncle.

When **bacteria** enter the skin through a hair follicle and multiply while producing toxins, they in turn are attacked by white blood cells, or **leukocytes** whose job it is to protect the body from such invasion. As the white blood cells consume the bacteria and destroy the infection, a pustule that comprises the center of a boil may form. The pustule is made up of white blood cells and cells destroyed by the bacteria that are trapped in the hair follicle. When the pustule pushes to the surface of the skin and erupts, the boil will drain and heal.

Boils are most often formed on the neck, face, or back, but they can be located anywhere on the skin. As they grow, they become red and hot; pressure exerted on surrounding nerves can cause considerable discomfort.

No attempt should be made to burst a boil prematurely by squeezing, as it may erupt under the skin and create new infection. Normally, the boil will mature on its own; however, frequent applications of a warm wet towel may hasten the process. Care should be taken to keep the area clean, especially after the boil erupts, in order to prevent spread of infection. A particularly severe boil or the presence of numerous boils may be symptomatic of other problems and should be referred to a physician. When a group of boils connects below the surface of the skin, the formation is called a **carbuncle**.

botulism

A type of food poisoning caused by a bacterium found in improperly canned or preserved food.

breastbone

In addition to the classic symptoms of food poisoning—nausea, vomiting, and abdominal cramps—toxin produced by the bacteria interferes with the transmission of nerve impulses and can cause irregularities in vision, followed by paralysis of the arms and difficulty breathing. Botulism can be fatal, so an early diagnosis and referral to a physician is critical.

breastbone

A bone at the front of the chest that travels downward from the collarbone and to which the ribs are attached; the sternum.

breast cancer

A malignant growth of the breast area that mainly attacks women over the age of 40. The exact cause of the cancer is not known—in some cases it seems to be hereditary, and there is evidence of increased risk among those whose diets include a significant amount of animal fat. Vitamin A and olive oil, on the other hand, have both shown in some studies to reduce the risk of breast cancer.

bronchitis

Inflammation of the bronchi, or air passages of the lung.

When the bronchial tubes, the air passages between the windpipe and the lungs, become infected and swollen, the glands in the mucous membrane that lines the tubes increase the secretion of mucus. The cough characteristic of bronchitis is an attempt to expel the excess fluid. In extreme cases, the infection may extend to the lungs and develop into *bronchopneumonia*.

Short term bronchitis, often following an attack of the common cold or influenza is called *acute bronchitis*. Bronchitis caused by repeated irritation from recurring infection, smoke, dust or other environmental effluence, is termed *chronic bronchitis*. Either condition is overcome only when the source of irritation has been removed.

Cigarette smoking is a primary cause of chronic bronchitis. Tobacco smoke interferes with the action of the hairlike fibers that push mucus from the lungs, allowing the mucus and irritants trapped by the mucus to remain in the lungs.

In addition to the characteristic cough, one who contracts acute bronchitis may experience flu–like symptoms: slight fever, a feeling of general malaise, aching muscles, etc. Treatment usually involves rest, steam inhalations and, if necessary, antibiotics to prevent further infection.

Chronic bronchitis often leads to permanent damage of the lungs and heart, and so should be left to the care of a physician.

brucellosis

An infection caused by the bacterium *Brucella* contracted from cattle, hogs or goats.

Also known as *undulant fever* or *Malta fever*, brucellosis is primarily contracted by persons in contact with animals or involved in meat processing, but it can also be transmitted in unpasteurized milk. Symptoms of the disease are similar to those for influenza: fever, headache, chills, and listlessness. The name *undulant fever* comes from a tendency of the condition to undulate, or move in waves, that is,

bubonic plague

bouts of the fever alternate with periods without symptoms.

bubonic plague

A highly contagious epidemic disease transmitted by the bite of infected rat fleas.

The name *bubonic* derives from a symptom of the disease: a bubo, or swelling, of lymph glands, especially in the armpit or groin. Similarly, a characteristic bleeding into the skin that causes dark blotches gave rise to the name *Black Death*.

The disease is now generally limited to unsanitary tropical areas, but there are occasional outbreaks in the western parts of the United States that are controlled by modern drugs.

bulimia

A disorder characterized by compulsive eating, often followed by self–induced vomiting. See also, *anorexia nervosa*.

bunion

An inflammation of the *bursa* at the first joint of the big toe. A bunion results from pressure against the toe that moves it laterally across the second toe and causes the base of the big toe to project outside the natural line of the foot, occurring most often among women who wear tight–fitting shoes.

Discomfort can usually be eased by relieving pressure on the toe. In some cases, a bunion has to be surgically removed.

bursa

A small sac that cushions the juncture between moving parts as bones, tendons, etc. The bursa contains a lubricating fluid that serves to eliminate

friction and promote smooth movement of the joints.
bursitis
Inflammation of a *bursa*. The swelling and tenderness from inflammation can cause such severe discomfort that movement is impossible.

Bursitis can be *chronic*, caused by repeated or constant stress on a joint, most commonly the elbow, shoulder or knee; or *acute*, caused by sudden trauma.

Immobilizing the joint may allow healing to take place, especially in the case of acute bursitis. Chronic bursitis is usually characterized by permanent damage frequently accompanied by calcium deposits that may render the joint immobile. Moist heat or cold compresses may ease the pain and aspirin or other pain relievers can also be effective. Surgery may be advised in extreme cases.

bypass
To skirt or circumvent, as a graft that allows the passage of blood around a clogged section of artery.

An artery narrowed by *atherosclerosis* places an added burden on the organ or tissue it services that can lead to further damage. In addition, there is the possibility that a blood clot will close the vessel completely, with catastrophic results. In many cases the problem can be resolved by grafting a section taken from another part of the body or by implanting a man–made device to circumvent the damaged section of the natural vessel.

cachexia
A weakened, emaciated state of the body caused by prolonged illness.

calcification
The abnormal accumulation of calcium salts in body tissue.

calculus
A solidified mass, as a stone, that may be formed in the kidneys, gallbladder or other organs of the body.

callus
A thickened growth of the skin; a callosity.

A callus is generally seen as protection to an area of the skin subjected to abnormal friction or pressure, as on parts of a laborer's hands or on the bottoms of the feet.

A callus may become so thick that the skin is inflexible and cracks, causing discomfort. In such a case, it may be necessary to remove the source of friction and consult a physician if discomfort is extreme. There are non–prescription medications that will soften the callosity, but removal at home should be considered carefully because of the danger of infection.

cancer
Any type of malignant growth.

Normal cells reproduce in a methodical manner in accordance with genetic coding; cancerous growth is uncontrolled, spreading throughout the body, destroying or replacing normal cells.

Cancer cells have the unique ability to propagate outside the organ where they originate; the cells may be carried in the blood or lymphatic channels to other parts of the body where they attack healthy tissue.

While there is no single preventative for cancer, the

risk of exposure may be lessened by avoiding known *carcinogens,* or cancer causing agents. Most cancer is treatable, so that early warning is also one of the best lines of defense. Symptoms to look for are: radical changes in bowel or bladder function; a wound that does not heal; unusual bleeding or discharge; chronic indigestion; a thickening lump anywhere on the body; any significant change in body function or formation.

candida
A fungal infection of the mouth, skin, intestines, or vagina caused by an imbalance of the body's natural fungi. In the mouth, candida causes pimples or *pustules*; on the skin it causes irritation often characterized by a rash; and in the vagina, itching accompanied by a cheese–like discharge. Treatment also varies; a physician should be consulted if infection is suspected.

canker sore
An ulcerated sore, usually of the lips or lining of the mouth.

Canker sores are not contagious, and may be induced by fever, allergy, or injury to the mouth, as from ill–fitting dentures.

capillaries
Extremely tiny blood vessels that connect the arteries and the veins.

carbohydrate
Any of a number of natural compounds that produce heat and energy, comprising the bulk of organic matter on earth.

carbuncle
A large boil formed from the interconnection of several boils.

Carbuncles cause severe pain associated with throbbing, possible fever and a feeling of malaise.

carcinogen
Any substance that promotes the formation of a cancerous growth.

carcinoma
Any of the malignant cancerous growths of the cells that line organs.

cardiology
The study of the heart and circulatory system especially diagnosis and treatment of disorders.

cardiopulmonary resuscitation See *CPR*.

cardiovascular system
The complex that circulates blood to all cells.

The cardiovascular system is made up of tubes called vessels, liquid contents called blood, and the pump which is the heart. These vessels are able to dilate and constrict. The size of the vessels is changed by signals transmitted through nerve pathways from the nervous system to the muscles in the blood vessel walls.

When the body is in its normal state there is enough blood to fill the system completely—approximately ten to twelve pints (for a person weighing 150 pounds). The pumping action of the heart supplies all parts of the body with blood.

Food and oxygen are transported to each part of the body and waste products are removed through this system.

carpal tunnel syndrome

Numbness, pain and weakness associated with compression of the *median nerve* at the wrist.

The finger tendons and the median nerve are contained in a tunnel formed by the carpal bones and the sturdy membrane that stretches over them. Any swelling of tissue within the tunnel can put pressure on the median nerve that controls the thumb, index finger, and middle finger.

Carpal tunnel syndrome may originate with pregnancy, a sprain or fracture of the wrist, arthritis, or any condition that tends to produce swelling or distortion of the wrist. The condition may be acquired or made worse by any activity that requires constant or repetitive twisting of the hand and wrist. Many cases are caused by long hours of working at a computer keyboard that requires keeping the hands at an unnatural angle.

The pain resulting from the condition has been known to run up the arm, into the shoulder and even the neck. Eventually, the sufferer may be unable to make a fist as the fingers weaken and the muscles atrophy.

The first step to recovery is to alleviate the pressure on the nerve by removing the cause; in severe cases, surgery may be necessary to prevent permanent damage. In extreme cases, that is, where treatment has been delayed, full recovery may not be possible.

carrier

An otherwise healthy individual who carries an infecting organism without evidence of symptoms, and who can infect others.

cartilage
The tough connective tissue between bones.
In the embryo, cartilage forms the skeleton that is later changed into bone. In the adult, the cartilage serves primarily to reduce friction in the joints and also functions as a cushion.

catabolism
The breaking down of complex substances by the body to provide energy; part of the total metabolic process. See also, *anabolism*.

cataleptic
One who suffers from periodic bouts of immobility characterized by muscular rigidity, an apparent suspension of awareness and, sometimes, loss of consciousness.

cataphasia
A condition characterized by frequent repetition of the same words or phrases.

cataract
A cloudiness or haziness of the lens of the eye that degrades vision.
In normal vision, the lens of the eye is clear and serves to direct light into the eye. When the lens becomes more or less opaque, the light is diffused, blurring the vision.
To correct the condition, the defective lens may be surgically removed, and replaced by an implant, special glasses or contact lenses.

catatonia
A phase of schizophrenia characterized by periods of muscular rigidity and withdrawal alternating with periods of agitation.

catheter
A hollow tube inserted into the body for the injection or withdrawal of fluids.

cat scratch fever
An ailment stemming from infection of a scratch, typically of the claw of a small animal, characterized by fever and chills, and swelling of the lymph glands.

cataracts
A clouding of the lens of the eye that interferes with vision. Cataracts can be removed by a relatively simple surgical procedure.

cerebral palsy
Any of a number of conditions marked by impaired muscle control.
Cerebral palsy is caused by nerve or brain damage, usually occurring around the time of birth.
Early signs of the condition may be convulsions, partial paralysis of face muscles, or slow development of motor functions, as sitting, crawling or standing. Later symptoms may range from a simple lack of coordination to the inability to move normally. The damage that causes cerebral palsy may also cause a number of other conditions, such as mental retardation, or learning and behavioral disorders.

charley horse
A painful cramp or stiffness caused by injury to a muscle when it is stretched suddenly, often caused by not warming up before strenuous exercise.

chemotherapy
Treatment of disease with the use of chemicals.

chest

The chest is formed by twenty–four ribs, twelve on each side, that are attached in the back to **vertebrae**. The seven upper pairs of ribs are attached to the **breastbone** in front by **cartilage**. The next three pairs of ribs are attached in front by a common cartilage to the seventh rib instead of the breastbone. The lower two pairs of ribs, known as the floating ribs, are not attached in front.

chest cavity

The chest cavity is cone–shaped, formed by the upper part of the spinal column, or backbone, at the back, the ribs on the sides, and the ribs and breastbone in front. The diaphragm, a thin, muscular partition at the bottom of the chest cavity, separates the chest cavity and the abdominal cavity.

The lungs and the heart occupy most of the chest cavity. In addition to the heart and the lungs, the chest cavity contains the esophagus or food pipe that extends from the back of the throat down through the diaphragm to the stomach, the trachea or windpipe that extends to the lungs, and several major blood vessels.

chickenpox

A highly contagious eruptive viral disease.

Chickenpox is so easily contracted that almost everyone is affected in childhood. The disease is spread by contact with an infected person or anything that has been contaminated by an infected person. The virus that causes chickenpox is the same virus that causes shingles, and chicken pox may also be contracted from a person who has shingles.

Chickenpox usually appears as an itchy rash of small red spots around the trunk. The spots quickly develop into larger blisters that spread throughout the body. Within a few days, the blisters burst and form a crust.

With few exceptions, the greatest danger from chickenpox is the potential for infection or scarring from aggressive rubbing of the itching blisters. Children may need to wear mittens, especially at night, to keep from scratching.

Treatment consists mainly of alleviating the symptoms, especially the annoying itch; applications of a soothing lotion may help. Daily warm baths will aid in clearing the rash and reduce the risk of infection. Aspirin should not be administered, because taking aspirin during a viral infection has been associated with bouts of *Reye's syndrome*, a far more serious infection.

Usually, one attack of chickenpox is enough to insure that an individual will be immune from further infection for life.

chilblain

Swelling of the skin due to exposure to cold.

The condition is seldom seen in areas where indoor heating and outdoor clothing are adequate to protect against winter cold and dampness.

Chilblains appear as itchy patches of red, swollen skin on the extremities that usually recede within a few days. A chronic condition can develop, however, with a discoloration of the skin accompanied by blisters that are painful and leave scars when they heal.

chill

Shivering, and a sense of being cold, often associated with a sudden increase in body temperature.

A chill often heralds the onset of infection, caused by a temporary disorder of the nerve centers that regulate body temperature. Typically, the chill develops as fever rises and may recur intermittently until the fever breaks.

chiropody

The science that deals with diseases, irregularities and injuries of the foot; see *podiatry*.

cholera

Any of various intestinal diseases transmitted in contaminated food or water, characterized by fever, vomiting, diarrhea, and dehydration.

cholesterol

A component of animal fat, blood, nerve tissue, and bile, some of which is necessary to a healthy body, but that may be harmful in excess, as in the formation of *atherosclerosis*.

See also, *lipoprotein*.

chorea

A nervous disorder characterized by uncontrollable involuntary actions of the body and limbs.

chromosomes

The body of genetic material contained in the nucleus of a cell, the basic unit that makes up all living things.

Chromosomes carry the genes that transmit the characteristics of a parent to a child, and through each cell throughout life, inasmuch as all cells in the body are created by division from the initial fertilized ovum, or egg.

cicatrix

The fibrous tissue remaining after a wound has healed; a scar.

circadian rhythm

Descriptive of the repetitive physiological processes of the body as they relate to the twenty–four hour cycle of the earth's rotation.

Everyone has a so–called *internal clock* that maintains a cyclic pattern of body processes coinciding more or less with a twenty–four hour day, as for the rising and falling of temperature, blood pressure, etc.

circulatory system

The functions and organs that carry blood to and from all parts of the body, consisting of the **heart** and **blood vessels**.

Through the blood vessels, **blood** is circulated throughout the body under pressure supplied by the pumping action of the heart.

cirrhosis

A disease of the liver in which healthy cells are destroyed and replaced by fibrous tissue.

Cirrhosis is the result of attempts by the liver to correct damage after sudden massive infection, as by acute **hepatitis**; over a period of months or years, as by chronic hepatitis or blockage of the bile ducts; or over a much longer period, as by alcohol abuse, the most common cause of cirrhosis.

Treatment for the condition mainly involves correcting the cause, as by removing the blockage or

claudication

discontinuing the ingestion of alcohol, then improving the diet to accommodate the damaged liver, as by large doses of vitamins and frequent small meals to reduce strain on the liver.

claudication

Limping or lameness, especially that caused by restriction of the flow of blood to the leg muscles, as by *atherosclerosis.*

claustrophobia

A morbid fear of being in a confined space or enclosed area.

cleft lip, cleft palate

A birth defect in which a part or all of the upper structure of the mouth is split.

If it is not corrected, the deformity can cause difficulty with speech and hearing; however, the most immediate problem may be feeding—the infant with a cleft lip or palate may not be able to suckle.

Often a special device or an appliance can be used to facilitate feeding until the time considered suitable by the physician to attempt corrective surgery.

clot See *blood clot.*

clubfoot

A birth defect in which the foot is turned inward or otherwise twisted.

Early correction may involve manipulation and the use of casts or other devices to gradually correct the position of the foot. Some surgery may be required to lengthen the Achilles tendon or correct the ankle joint. If early attempts at correction are not successful, or not undertaken, extensive surgery may be required.

coagulation
The transformation of a liquid into a soft, congealed mass, as in clotting.

cocaine
A narcotic used as a local anesthetic, effective when applied to mucous membrane, that is addictive when inhaled.
See also, *codeine*.

coccyx
A small bone that forms the lower extremity of the spinal column.

codeine
An opium derivative, used for the relief of pain, similar to morphine, but not as addictive.

cod-liver oil
Fish oil that is rich in vitamins A and D, often taken as a dietary supplement.

cold sore
A viral infection that causes small blisters to appear about the area of the mouth, usually following an illness accompanied by fever.

colostomy
A surgical procedure in which an opening is created in the wall of the abdomen and joined to an opening in the large intestine to allow the elimination of body waste.
A colostomy may be created to correct a condition caused by obstruction or disease.
Waste discharged through the opening is collected in a disposable bag that must be changed by the wearer. Once the diet is properly regulated, the colostomy causes little restriction of normal activities.

compress
A pad, often of cloth, used to apply heat, moisture, or medication.

compulsion
An irresistible desire, often irrational and repetitive, to do something.

concretion
A hard, inorganic mass in the body, as a kidney stone; a calculus.

concussion
An injury to the brain caused by sudden shock, as a sharp blow to the head.

A simple concussion, brought about by the brain striking the inside of the skull, may result in bruising brain tissue, bleeding inside the skull, and possible loss of consciousness.

Unconsciousness may last a few minutes or a few hours; a longer period usually indicates more serious damage. Other symptoms of a concussion are feelings of nausea, dizziness, and headache that may last for several days. There may also be a loss of memory for a period just prior to the injury until several hours after.

Any signs of more serious injury, as an open wound, partial paralysis anywhere in the body or sharply dilated pupils should be referred to a physician.

Normally, rest is all that is required for recuperation. The victim should relax, avoid any medication stronger than aspirin and, if vomiting occurs, avoid solid food. Sleep ought to be postponed for several hours to be certain that no unusual symptoms arise and, once allowed to sleep, the victim should be awakened every two hours to give his or her name and location so as to confirm that there are no complications.

Consult a physician if a headache grows more severe, vision becomes blurred or there is any other abnormality of the eyes, and in case of spasms or staggering.

congenital
Existing from birth; descriptive of a condition present at birth and that is not hereditary.

congestion
An abnormal accumulation of body fluid, especially one that tends to clog.

conjunctivitis
An inflammation of the conjunctiva, the membrane that covers the outer surface of the eyeball and lines the inner surface of the eyelid.

Conjunctivitis is often caused by the invasion of microorganisms and may be contracted by dust, smoke, or chemicals. Those with allergies are often victims.

The condition is characterized by redness of the eye, burning or itching, and a sensitivity to light. There is often periodic tearing and a discharge of pus.

Treatment varies with the cause of the disease and its severity. The eye should be rested and protected from bright light as much as possible; if eyelids are held closed by dry discharge, the hardened matter can be softened by gently bathing the eyes in warm water. Care should be taken to isolate handkerchiefs, towels, etc. used by the subject, as conjunctivitis is highly contagious.

connective tissue
Fibrous tissue that serves to connect the cells and support the organs of the body.

contact dermatitis
An inflammation of the skin caused by direct contact with an irritant.

Contact dermatitis may be caused by any of a number of substances, such as detergent, hair coloring, cosmetics, household cleaners, or by plants, such as poison ivy and poison oak.

Contact with an irritant to which the subject is sensitive may cause redness, swelling, blistering, burning, itching, or tenderness in the area of contact.

Identifying the offending substance may be a simple process of elimination or it may require the assistance of a doctor who can test for allergies. The infection may clear when the substance is avoided; more severe cases should be referred to a doctor for medication.

contagion
The spread of disease, directly or indirectly, from one person to another.

contaminated
Descriptive of that which is unclean, often in reference to food or water infected by bacteria.

contusion
A bruise or injury that does not break the skin.

convulsion
Sudden, involuntary contractions or spasms of the muscles.

corns See *callus*.

coronary bypass See *bypass*.
coronary heart disease See *atherosclerosis*.
corticosteroids
Any of the hormones produced in the cortex of the adrenal glands.
More than 30 corticosteroids regulate essential processes in the body.
One group, the mineralocorticoids, help maintain the salt and water balance in the body. A second group, the glucocorticoids, help regulate the use of sugars and proteins. The third group, androgens, stimulate the development of secondary male sex characteristics.
cough
Sudden, noisy expulsion of air from the lungs.
Coughing is a defensive reflex that clears the lungs of excess mucus or irritating matter. The cough will persist as long as the condition that causes it, but it may be suppressed by soothing liquids or drugs that act on the cough reflex.
CPR
CardioPulmonary Resuscitation; the use of artificial ventilation, that is, mouth–to–mouth breathing and external heart compression, to revive one who has suffered cardiac arrest.
cretinism
A severe congenital thyroid deficiency.
The infant suffering from cretinism exhibits retarded physical and mental development that, if diagnosed early, may be treated and cured.
crib death
The sudden, unexplained, death of an apparently

croup

healthy infant; sudden infant death syndrome or
SIDS.

croup

An inflammation of the larynx.

A condition mostly confined to children, the croup
causes swelling of the larynx, or voice box, so that
breathing becomes difficult. A characteristic barking
cough is the result of air forced through the swollen
larynx. Breathing may be further impaired if mucus
blocks the windpipe and bronchi that connect to the
lungs. Immediate medical attention is critical, because the swelling may close off the passage completely.

In the meantime, calm the child—an attack of croup
is frightening and fear can only make the symptoms
worse. If possible, sit in a bathroom with the hot
shower running—the warm, moist air should ease
the symptoms. Similar results may be obtained with
the use of a humidifier or by breathing over a container of hot water with a tent fashioned from a
towel over the head; however, resting in a parent's
arms in the steamy atmosphere of a bathroom is
probably most soothing.

cyclamate

A sugar substitute banned from use in the U.S. after
studies revealed that it caused cancer in laboratory
animals.

cyst

An abnormal sac containing liquid or semiliquid
waste material.

Cysts often do not cause symptoms and are therefore not treated; one that causes pressure or other

problems may be surgically removed.

cystic fibrosis

A hereditary disease that affects mainly the respiratory system and sweat glands, and that usually develops during childhood. Cystic fibrosis is distinguished by the production of abnormally thick sticky mucus that clogs air passages causing frequent respiratory infections.

A child with cystic fibrosis will exhibit a variety of symptoms including chronic coughing and fever, difficulty in breathing, and a poor appetite. The disease can often be treated at home with a special diet and antibiotics.

decortication

Removal of the outer layer of an organ.

defibrillation

A technique to correct fibrillation, an abnormal heartbeat.

Fibrillation is commonly caused by a heart attack, when part of the heart quivers or acts independently of the normal heartbeat. The heart is not then able to pump blood through the body and death will result if the condition is not corrected.

Protracted exposure to the cold or a severe electrical shock can also cause fibrillation.

degenerative joint disease See *osteoarthritis*.

dehydration

Loss of water from the body; the condition produced by loss of water or deprivation of water from body tissue.

Dehydration may be caused by the inability to take in water due to illness or disease, or by loss of water

delirium

from vomiting, diarrhea, uncontrolled secretion of urine, or excessive sweating.

A serious side affect of dehydration is the critical loss of salt from the body. Unchecked dehydration may result in death in a matter of days.

delirium

A temporary mental disorder characterized by excitement, confusion and hallucinations.

Delirium may be brought on by any of a number of traumatic conditions, as by infection, drugs, withdrawal of certain drugs or alcohol, high fever, etc.

Condition of the subject may undergo abrupt radical change with varying frequency, as from a state of agitated restlessness to one of serenity and comprehension.

delirium tremens *(DT's)*

Disordered perception brought on by trauma associated with alcoholism.

Delirium tremens may be triggered by a bout of excessive alcohol consumption, by the consumption of alcohol in conjunction with other drugs, even those that would be otherwise innocuous, or by withdrawal of alcohol after a period of excess consumption.

The victim may suffer distinctive tremors, frightening hallucinations, rapid pulse, periods of profuse sweating, an overwhelming feeling of terror, extreme agitation.

delusion

A belief maintained in spite of irrefutable evidence to the contrary.

Delusion may be part of a psychotic episode in

which perception is altered to cause irrational interpretation of an ordinary event. In such cases, there may not be even a remote connection between the event and the interpretation.

On another level, delusion may be formed from hallucination or an elaborate scheme of rationalization that, although connected, has no basis in reality.

Delusion may also be related to depression, as in feelings of hypochondria or guilt, where the subject has negative feelings relating to personal condition, fortunes, or worthiness that are not supported in fact.

dementia

Mental impairment or deficiency caused by injury or disease.

Dementia may be associated with senility, *Alzheimer's disease*, a blood clot or tumor of the brain, etc.

A loss of memory, especially for recent events, is the most common symptom of dementia. The condition can progress to a stage where the subject suffers severe degradation or total destruction of intellectual powers, deprivation of emotional control, and a complete personality transformation.

See also, *amentia*.

dentistry

The work of one whose profession is the care of the teeth and the surrounding tissue.

Dentistry involves the diagnosis and treatment of the diseases and disorders of the mouth, as well as prevention of those conditions.

Routine dental care is normally provided by a

dermatitis

general practitioner who is qualified to recommend a specialist, if one is needed. Among the specialized fields of dentistry are: *orthodontia,* concerned with the straightening of teeth; *periodontia,* that deals with diseases of the gums; *prosthodontia,* the replacement of missing teeth; *endodontia,* focusing on diseases of the pulp and root canal surgery; and *exodontia,* dealing with the extraction of teeth.

dermatitis

Any inflammation of the skin.

Dermatitis may be caused by any of a number of substances, such as detergent, hair coloring, cosmetics, or household cleaners; by plants, such as poison ivy and poison oak; or by ingesting certain foods or medications, etc.

Contact with an irritant to which the subject is sensitive may cause redness, swelling, blistering, burning, itching, or tenderness in the area of contact.

Identifying an offending substance may be a simple process of elimination or it may require the assistance of a doctor to run tests for allergies. The infection may clear when the substance is avoided; more severe cases can require medication.

Some forms of dermatitis are a secondary symptom of diseases affecting other parts of the body and others, such as *exfoliative dermatitis* that causes the shedding of skin and hair, must be referred to a physician for proper diagnosis and cure.

dermatology

The study of diseases and disorders of the skin.

Because of the relationship between diseases of the

skin and allergies or other diseases (see **dermatitis**), the dermatologist must have a thorough knowledge of diseases that relate to dermatitis and of allergies.

deviated septum

An internal disorder in which the membrane that separates the nostrils is bent to one side. One may be born with a deviated septum or it may be caused by injury.

Often there is no external indication of the deviation and it need be treated only if it poses a health problem such as difficulty in breathing, or nasal congestion that leads to recurring infections. Treatment for a troublesome deviated septum involves relatively simple corrective surgery.

diabetes mellitus

A condition in which the body is not able to satisfactorily process ingested sugar.

Body and brain cells need many different types of nourishment, one of which is sugar. The circulatory system carries sugar and transfers it to the cells with the aid of a chemical substance called insulin. The pancreas, located in the abdominal cavity, manufactures insulin. When the insulin production and sugar are in balance, the body functions normally. An individual suffering from a reduction in the production of insulin is said to have diabetes mellitus.

As a result of this imbalance, the body is adversely affected; however, a great many diabetics lead healthy, normal lives through a program of balanced diet and medication. When the diabetic's condition is not controlled, certain disorders may occur.

diabetic coma

The major adverse reactions to insulin imbalance are *diabetic coma* and *insulin shock*.

diabetic coma

A state of stupor or lethargy leading to coma, brought on by an inadequate supply of insulin.

This imbalance that triggers diabetic coma is generally due to a diabetic not taking the proper medication; a diabetic ingesting more sugar than the available insulin can accommodate; a person contracting an infection that affects insulin production; or sustained vomiting or fluid loss.

The signs of someone progressing into diabetic coma are warm and dry skin, sunken eyes, rapid and labored breathing, rapid and weak pulse, excessive urination accompanied by extreme thirst, nausea and vomiting, abdominal pain, a state of confusion and disorientation that is similar to drunkenness. Eventually the condition leads to a coma state, thus the term *diabetic coma*.

diagnosis

The process of identifying a disease by careful examination of symptoms.

dialysis

The process of removing waste matter and maintaining the electrolyte balance of the blood by diffusion.

Normally, dialysis is performed by the kidneys. One who suffers kidney failure, whether temporary or permanent, must have the blood cleansed by the use of an artificial kidney machine. The blood from a tube implanted in an artery is circulated through the machine where it comes in contact with a thin membrane that separates the blood from a solution containing a precise concentration of electrolytes. By the process of osmosis, the tendency of certain fluids to diffuse through a membrane from a stronger to a weaker solution, the wastes are passed through the membrane to the solution and electrolytes are passed from the solution to the blood. The blood cells, too large to pass through the membrane, are not affected and the revitalized blood is returned to the subject's body through a tube implanted in a vein.

diaphragm
The muscular partition in the body that separates the chest cavity and the abdominal cavity.

diarrhea
The frequent and excessive discharging of watery feces.

Diarrhea can be caused by a number of conditions such as food poisoning, an allergic reaction to food or drugs, an infection of the gastrointestinal tract, or disease. Most bouts of diarrhea last only a short time as the body rids itself of contaminate matter. If the diarrhea persists more than a few hours, an over–the–counter preparation may help.

A major complication associated with an incidence of diarrhea is the possibility of dehydration, especially in small children.

If the condition persists or is accompanied by other symptoms such as fever, abdominal pain, or vomiting, a physician should be consulted.

dietary fiber See *fiber*.

digestion
The process of breaking down food into those

substances that can be used by the body and those that are to be discharged as waste.

Digestion begins in the mouth where food is ground by the teeth and mixed with saliva. The saliva both moistens food for easier passage, and begins the breakdown of starches. The food is passed down the throat, through the esophagus and into the stomach, at which point it is combined with digestive juices to partly liquefy it for passage into the small intestine. In the duodenum, the first section of the small intestine, bile from the liver aids in the absorption of fat and digestive juices from the pancreas further facilitate the digestion and absorption of food. Anything that is not absorbed into the bloodstream from the small intestine is passed on to the large intestine for discharge from the body.

diphtheria

An acute, highly contagious disease that affects the tonsils, airways and larynx.

Diphtheria bacteria destroy the outer layer of mucous membrane in the throat or larynx. The principal mark of the disease is a grayish membrane over the throat formed from dead cells, bacteria, etc.

Diphtheria is transmitted by drops of moisture from the nose and throat of an infected person, often a carrier who is not aware of the presence of the disease.

Symptoms of the disease include sore throat, hoarseness, a rasping cough and fever. Children may be nauseous, with chills and a headache in addition to other symptoms. The characteristic membrane may vary in color or not appear at all;

however, if it does form, it may detach and block off the victim's air supply. Because of the danger, sufferers need to be hospitalized where they can recuperate under close supervision.

The disease may be complicated by inflammation of the heart muscles or nerves.

dislocation

Twisting out of normal position, as a bone.

Where two or more bones come together to form a joint, they are held in place by bands of strong, fibrous tissue called ligaments. Of the three types of joint, those that are immovable, those with limited motion, and those that are freely movable, the freely movable joints—those of the lower jaw, the shoulders, the elbows, the wrists, the fingers, the hips, the knees, the ankles, and the toes, are the ones most commonly dislocated.

When one or more of the bones forming a joint slip out of normal position, the ligaments holding the bones are stretched and sometimes torn loose. Fractures are often associated with dislocations. Dislocation may result from force applied at or near the joint, a sudden muscular contraction, twisting strains on joint ligaments, or a fall where the force of landing is transferred to a joint.

Some general symptoms of dislocations are a rigidity and loss of function, deformity, pain, swelling, tenderness, and discoloration. Resetting a dislocation is not a trivial matter—the victim should be placed in a doctor's care as quickly as possible.

diverticulosis, diverticulitis

A *diverticulum* is a small sac or pouch; *diverticulosis*

is the existence of *diverticula* (plural form of diverticulum) on the wall of the bowel.; *diverticulitis* is an inflammation of the diverticula.

It is possible, though not proven, that diverticula are formed when a lack of roughage in the diet causes the muscle layer in the wall of the colon to overwork or when those muscles are weakened by age, so that pressure in the colon forces the intestinal lining through the weak spots in the wall. Generally, diverticulosis exhibits no symptoms; however, waste matter may become trapped in the diverticula and reduce the flow of blood to the walls, paving the way for diverticulitis.

In addition to discomfort and pain in the abdomen, diverticulitis may lead to the formation of a fistula, or unnatural channel, between the colon and the bladder or another organ, infecting it as well.

DNA, RNA

DNA is deoxyribonucleic acid, the basic component of living tissue that holds the genetic information to insure the inheritance and transmission of chromosomes and genes

RNA is ribonucleic acid, that carries the genetic information from DNA for the synthesis of protein in the cell.

DT's See delirium tremens

duodenal ulcer

An ulcer, or open sore affecting the duodenum, the first section of the small intestine.

A *peptic ulcer* is an infection in any part of the digestive tract exposed to pepsin, a digestive juice. A *duodenal ulcer* is a type of peptic ulcer occurring in the duodenum when its lining is attacked by the action of digestive juices to which it is normally impervious.

Though unconfirmed, the cause of the ulcer may be excessive secretions of digestive juices by the stomach brought about by diet or medication.

The ulcer may remain undetected as for lack of symptoms, but usually will cause some discomfort of the abdomen, such as a burning sensation, within an hour of two of eating. The presence of the ulcer needs to be confirmed by a physician who can prescribe medication, but treatment may simply require avoiding foods that cause distress as well as those that stimulate the secretion of digestive fluids, such as caffeinated beverages and alcohol

dysentery

An inflammation of the colon characterized by pain, cramps and diarrhea.

The infection, caused by bacteria, *bacillary dysentery,* or amoebae, *amoebic dysentery*, is spread through poor hygiene, as by contaminated food.

dyslexia

Any of a number of reading, writing or learning disorders in one who is otherwise of normal intelligence.

Most symptoms relate to a lack of directional or positional sense in that letters in a word or words in a sentence may be read or written out of their normal order, or there may be difficulty matching names with their respective images.

dyspepsia

Indigestion; impaired digestion.

dysphagia

Belching, stomach pains, a feeling that the stomach is overfull, a sour taste, and even nausea, are all signs of indigestion, usually brought about by poor dietary habits. Ingesting fatty foods, rich foods, spicy foods, an excess of alcohol, or irregular meals all make one a prime candidate for dyspepsia.

Dyspepsia is quite common and seldom causes more than temporary discomfort; however, if it is chronic, that is, occurs regularly after meals or frequently causes sleep to be interrupted, it may be warning of a more serious condition.

dysphagia

Difficulty in swallowing.

There are a number of conditions that can cause dysphagia, such as blockage, muscular spasms, ulcers, diverticulum (small sac or pouches on the esophagus), infection, or cancer.

A physician should be consulted promptly if the condition persists.

E. coli

One of a number of strains of rod–shaped bacteria that live in the intestinal tracts of humans and other animals. Many of the strains are harmless, but a notable exception is a one that can contaminate beef. Although illness from contaminated beef is rare, it has been suggested that all meat, and especially ground beef, be cooked until it is no longer pink.

eczema

Any inflammatory disease of the skin.

Eczema may manifest itself in redness, burning or itching, blistering, the discharge of serous matter, and crusts or scabs.

edema

Swelling caused by the accumulation of fluid in the tissues.

elective surgery

Surgery to correct a condition that is not life threatening, such as plastic surgery.

embolism

Blockage of a blood vessel by an obstruction called an embolus.

Blockage of a blood vessel by an obstruction called an embolus.

A common form of embolus is a blood clot or plaque from a clogged artery or heart valve. An air embolus may develop if an excessive amount of air is admitted during an intravenous injection, during surgery, or in moving between an area of high pressure and an area of lower pressure; see *bends*.

An embolism reduces the supply of blood to the area where it occurs causing tissue damage. Discomfort or pain may be the main symptom of an embolism with others depending on the location, as an embolism in a brain artery that emulates the symptoms of a *stroke*.

emphysema

A lung condition in which the air spaces in the lungs are enlarged.

Emphysema often develops from the inflammation, swelling and excessive mucus production associated with bronchitis or other disease that traps air in the lungs. The result is a loss of effectiveness in moving air in and out of the lungs, putting extra strain on the heart.

Emphysema is characterized by shortness of breath. Difficulty in breathing may be accompanied by a persisting, painful cough. Sufferers of emphysema tire quite easily, largely a result of the energy required just to get enough air.

encephalitis

Inflammation of the brain.

Encephalitis may be caused by bacteria or parasites, but most commonly is the result of a virus, either as a direct effect or complication from an infection.

Some of the viruses are carried by mosquitoes while others are associated with childhood diseases, as measles, mumps, or chicken pox—children are the main victims of the disease.

endocarditis

Inflammation of the valves or lining of the heart.

endocrinology

The study of the endocrine system and its functions as well as the diagnosis and treatment of its disorders.

The endocrine system is comprised of the glands that secrete vital hormones into the bloodstream, including the pituitary, adrenal, thyroid, pancreas, ovaries, and testes.

The hormones secreted by these glands travel throughout the body to control and combine a number of body functions. Growth abnormalities, diabetes and other diseases may be attributed to disorders of the endocrine system.

enteritis

Inflammation of the intestinal tract.

Enteritis is most commonly found as a bacterial or viral infection in the small intestine as the result of the consumption of contaminated food or water.

epidemiology

The study of the onset, recurrence, pattern of distribution, and control of disease.

Epidemiology deals with the communication of disease in general, the relationship between certain diseases and the conditions under which they flourish, and means of prevention, such as vaccines.

The epidemiologist is also concerned with non-infectious diseases that are widespread or of questionable origin, such as the relationship between certain illnesses and environmental pollution, or toxic substances in foods or other products.

epilepsy

A neurological disorder that causes recurring seizures.

Commonly, epilepsy has no apparent cause, although in some cases it may be traced to a source, such as a tumor that forms pressure on the brain, an injury to the brain, or disorder caused by drugs.

Seizures may be so mild as to go virtually unnoticed or so severe that they can result in serious harm. The subject may be aware of an impending seizure by a tingling sensation in the extremities accompanied by distortion in the senses of sight and smell, as be seeing flashing lights and perceiving bad odors. The seizure may be marked by sitting motionless, as though daydreaming; moving or behaving in a repetitive or inappropriate manner; or by convulsions. A convulsive attack may cause the subject to cry out, stiffen and fall unconscious, lose urinary and bowel control, or exhibit jerking, spastic or thrashing movements. Convulsions are usually followed by deep sleep and no recollection of the seizure.

The epileptic may be treated by correcting any physical disorder and prescribing medication. Non–medical treatment is limited to monitoring the seizure: make the subject comfortable by loosening clothing if necessary or placing a pillow under the head; protect the subject from inhaling vomit or otherwise suffocating; make no attempt to pry open the mouth or insert anything into the mouth of a person who is having a convulsion.

Epilepsy cannot be prevented, but the seizures may be controlled by medication, allowing the epileptic to lead a normal life.

esophagus

The food pipe, that extends from the throat, through the chest, ending at the stomach.

excretory systems

Those parts of the body concerned with the separation and elimination of waste products.

Several different systems serve to eliminate waste products that enter the body or are formed within it. The residue of food taken into the digestive system, mainly indigestible materials, together with secretions from various glands emptying into the intestines, is gathered in the lower portion of the large intestine and eliminated through the rectum as feces.

Surplus water, carrying dissolved salts that are excess in the system or form a waste product, is extracted by the kidneys, collected in the bladder, and expelled as urine.

Carbon dioxide and certain volatile products carried by the blood are exchanged in the lungs for oxygen and pass from the body in exhaled air.

The skin contains many small organs known as sweat glands that are important in eliminating heat, excess fluid, and dissolved waste products from the body.

extrasystole

An abnormal contraction of the heart.

Normally, the heart beats in a regular rhythm; an extrasystole is a contraction of the heart caused by a signal emanating from somewhere other than the heart's natural pacemaker.

The extrasystole may be detected as a skip, flutter, or extra beat. It may be experienced periodically, triggered by stress or excitement, or it may be recurring, as a symptom of heart disease or reaction to drugs. Whether the extrasystole is a matter for concern depends on its cause, frequency, and the general health of the subject, for example triggered by stress in one with a heart condition, the extrasystole may lead to more serious problems. Prolonged symptoms, as well, should be referred to a physician.

extremities

Descriptive of arms and legs including their joining to the trunk of the body.

The *upper extremity* consists of thirty–two bones. The collarbone is a long bone, the inner end of which is attached to the breastbone and the outer end is attached to the shoulder blade at the shoulder joint. The collarbone lies just in front of and above the first rib. The shoulder blade is a flat triangular bone which lies at the upper and outer part of the back of the chest and forms part of the shoulder joint. The arm bone extends from the shoulder to the elbow. The two bones of the forearm extend from the elbow to the wrist. There are eight wrist bones, five bones in the palm of the hand, and fourteen finger bones, two in the thumb and three in each finger.

The *lower extremity* consists of thirty bones. The thigh bone, the longest and strongest bone in the body, extends from the hip joint to the knee; its upper end is rounded to fit into the socket in the pelvis, and its lower end broadens out to help form part of the knee joint. This flat triangular bone can be felt in front of the knee joint. The two bones in the leg extend from the knee joint to the ankle. There are seven bones in the ankle and back part of the foot, five long bones in the front part of the foot, and fourteen toe bones.

febrile
Descriptive of body temperature that is above normal; feverish.

fever blisters
An eruption about the mouth accompanying a cold or fever; cold sore or herpes simplex.

fiber
A form of indigestible plant matter. The digestive system cannot break down dietary fiber and although it passes through the body without being absorbed, it plays an important role in digestion.

Certain types of fiber combine with water to ease the passage of material through the colon; others are purported to lower cholesterol levels.

Among the best sources of fiber are fruits, vegetables, legumes, and unprocessed grain in bread and cereal.

fistula

An abnormal duct or passageway in the body.

A fistula may be congenital or the complication of an infection.

folliculitis

An infection of a follicle or follicles, especially hair follicles. Commonly, folliculitis results from bacteria entering a hair follicle on the face when shaving, then spreads to the surrounding area.

food allergy

Excessive sensitivity to a particular food that is otherwise considered safe to eat.

A food allergy exists when the immune system reacts to a particular food or to a substance in the food by manufacturing antibodies. The foods that most commonly trigger an immune system reaction are dairy products, seafood, chocolate, tomatoes, strawberries, and citrus fruits.

A food reaction is usually manifested by digestive disorders, as cramps, nausea, vomiting, or diarrhea; however, hives, rash, nasal congestion, headache, or *anaphylactic shock* may also be symptoms.

When a food allergy is suspected, the offending substance can often be pinpointed by the process of elimination, that is, sampling or excluding foods one at a time to determine if symptoms recur. This can

food poisoning

also be done by maintaining a record of all foods eaten over a period of time and observing the reaction or lack of reaction, as sensitivity may be triggered by consuming certain foods in combination.

food poisoning

Acute distress caused by food containing toxins or bacteria.

Food poisoning is the result of ingesting a subsistence that in its natural state contains poison, as certain wild mushrooms and plants, or one that has been contaminated, as food that has been improperly stored.

Cramps, diarrhea and vomiting are most commonly associated with food poisoning, but symptoms in some cases may be more severe, causing difficulty in breathing, blurred vision or paralysis. Any symptoms that are excessive or that persevere should be treated by a physician.

fracture

Any break or crack in a bone.

Fractures can be divided into two classifications:

an open, or compound fracture in which the bone is broken and an open wound is present often with the end of the broken bone protruding from the wound;

a closed, or simple fracture in which no open wound is present, but there is a broken or cracked bone.

Broken bones, especially the long bones of the upper and lower extremities, often have sharp, sawtooth edges so that even slight movement may cause the sharp edges to cut into blood vessels, nerves, or muscles. Careless or improper movement can convert a closed fracture into an open fracture, causing

damage to surrounding blood vessels or nerves
If the broken ends of the bone extend through an
open wound, there is little doubt that the victim has
suffered a fracture; however, the bone does not always extend through the skin, so it is well to be able
to recognize other signs that a fracture exists, such
as pain or tenderness in the area, deformity or irregularity of the affected area, loss of function, discoloration, and swelling.
Any fracture or suspected fracture should be referred to a physician, as improper healing can have
serious consequences.

friable
Descriptive of that which is easily pulverized.

frostbite
Tissue damage caused by extreme cold.
Frostbite is most likely to occur when the wind is
blowing, rapidly drawing heat from the body. The
nose, cheeks, ears, toes, and fingers are the body
parts most frequently frostbitten. As a result of exposure to cold, the blood vessels constrict causing
the blood supply to the chilled parts to decrease and
depriving the tissues of the warmth they need.
The signs and symptoms of frostbite are not always
apparent to the sufferer, because frostbite has a
numbing effect.
Frostbite goes through the following stages: the affected area will feel numb; the skin turns red, then
dead white or blue–white; eventually the skin and
underlying tissue is firm to the touch.
Treatment for the early stage of frostbite involves
placing the affected part close to the body for

warmth without rubbing. In the later stages, there is severe, perhaps permanent, damage to the tissue so that it must not be rubbed, it should be lightly covered for protection, and heat should not be applied. The subject should seek medical attention immediately; if skin is frozen, it should remain so until the subject is hospitalized as thawing is extremely painful. Avoid anything that may constrict blood vessels, such as smoking, coffee, tea or hot chocolate.

fulminating
Descriptive of the onset of a disease that is rapid and severe.

furuncle See *boil*.

gallstones
Hardened masses formed in the gallbladder or in the bile duct leading from the gallbladder to the small intestine.

Gallstones, formed from cholesterol, blood, bile, and other substances, may produce no symptoms or they can cause pain in the abdomen, indigestion, especially after eating fatty foods, or nausea. Sometimes the stones pass into the intestine and are excreted.

If the stones become trapped in the bile duct, the pain is much more severe and may be accompanied by chills, fever, vomiting and jaundice, especially if the flow of bile is blocked.

gangrene
Death of body tissue.

Gangrene is usually caused by a reduction or complete absence of blood to a section of tissue, although bacterial infection that destroys tissue may play a critical part in its formation.

Gangrene may be the result of burns, freezing, physical injury, a blood clot, bacteria or any other condition that interferes with the flow of blood and destroys tissue.

gastritis

Inflammation of the stomach lining.

gastroenteritis

Inflammation of the lining of the stomach and intestines.

Gastroenteritis is often the result of infection by bacteria or virus, but may also be caused by reaction to certain foods or drugs, by food poisoning, or by over consumption of alcohol.

The onset of gastroenteritis may be signaled by a feeling of discomfort in the abdomen, gas pains, cramps, nausea or diarrhea. Usually all that is required to alleviate the symptoms is rest, plenty of liquids and a temporary bland diet. Medical care may be required if symptoms persist in order to rule out a more serious condition.

Excessive vomiting and diarrhea may lead to dehydration that also requires medical attention, especially for infants.

gastroenterology

The branch of medicine that deals with the study, diagnosis and treatment of diseases and disorders of the stomach and intestines.

gene

Any of the units that occur in the chromosome and carry the traits that are passed on from parent to child

generic
Of a class or group—descriptive of drugs and other products that are prescribed and sold by their scientific name; a product that tends to be less expensive than one sold by brand name.

genetic
Descriptive of characteristics that may be inherited; distinctive from *congenital*, that is dating from birth.

genetic disorder
A disease or malformation that may be passed from one generation to another.

In some cases, the link is clearly established, as when a conditions is associated with a particular chromosome; in others, the association is established only by observation, as the tendency of a particular condition to occur in succeeding generations of a family.

germ
Generally, a reference to those microorganisms, especially bacteria, that are capable of producing disease.

German measles
A mild, contagious, viral infection; rubella.

The most serious problem associated with German measles is the likelihood of birth defect when the virus has been contracted during pregnancy.

gerontology
The study of the aging process and the diseases and disabilities associated with it.

giardiasis
A parasitic infection of the small intestine caused mainly by ingesting contaminated water.

gingivitis
Inflammation of the gums.

Gingivitis is usually due to a combination of poor diet and poor dental hygiene, although it may be caused by vitamin deficiency or as a complication of a disease.

The discomfort and minor bleeding associated with gingivitis may be alleviated by reducing the intake of sugar and alcohol, increasing the intake of vitamin C, and improving dental hygiene. In some cases, it is necessary for a dental surgeon to cut away damaged portions of the gum.

gland
Any organ that secretes a substance to be used elsewhere in the body.

glaucoma
A disorder of the eye caused by increased pressure within the eyeball.

Normally, fluid in the eyeball is under slight pressure that is carefully regulated. When fluid fails to drain and maintain a constant pressure, the buildup causes damage to the structure.

Glaucoma may be linked to other diseases of the eye or to the use of certain drugs.

Acute glaucoma is rare. The symptoms are so intense as to be impossible to ignore: extreme pain and a sudden blurring of vision. Deterioration by chronic glaucoma, on the other hand, is free of pain and so very gradual that it may go unnoticed for a long time. Initially, there may be some loss of peripheral vision without any other symptoms, followed by blurred vision, difficulty in adjusting to

globulin

bright lights or darkness, and slight pain around the eye, symptoms that may be sporadic.

Most eye examinations include a check for glaucoma in order to catch it in the early stages when it can be treated most effectively.

globulin

Any of several simple proteins that comprise one of the two major protein groups of the blood, insoluble in water. See also, *albumin.*

glossitis

Inflammation of the tongue.

Glossitis may be specific, as an injury to the tongue or it may be symptomatic of another disorder, as a disease or vitamin deficiency.

The symptoms of glossitis vary considerably, depending on the cause. Some of the manifestations are redness, swelling, white patches, and ulcers.

Severe acute glossitis produced by infection, burns, or injury can bring about pain and swelling that causes the tongue to project into the throat, obstructing the airway. In severe cases, chewing, swallowing, or speaking may be impaired.

glucose

A form of sugar found naturally in honey, fruit, and in the blood.

glycemia

The presence of sugar in the blood. See also *hyperglycemia*, *hypoglycemia.*

glycogen

A form of carbohydrate, found mainly in the muscles and in the liver, that is changed into glucose to meet the body's demands.

goiter

Enlargement of the thyroid gland that appears as a swelling at the side or front of the neck.

Goiter may be caused by a diet deficient in the iodine necessary for the production of thyroid hormone; by an excess of foods that inhibit the production of thyroid hormone, as cabbage or soya; or by a cause unknown.

The swelling is the result of a futile attempt by the gland to produce more hormone by enlarging the cells within the gland.

gout

Inflammation of a joint caused by excess uric acid in the bloodstream.

Gout is the result of the body's inability to properly process uric acid, a chemical normally found in the blood and urine. Excess uric acid may crystallize and be deposited in the skin, joints and kidneys.

An attack of gout is the body's response to the crystal deposits. The initial attack is usually concentrated in a single joint; subsequent attacks may involve several joints. Attacks are very painful and the area becomes extremely sensitive, followed by redness, warmth and swelling.

A physician should be consulted for treatment, even when the symptoms disappear within a day or two, because the condition tends to reappear with increasing frequency, duration, and severity.

graft

Living tissue that is taken from a body to be surgically implanted in another part of the body or in another body. See also *transplant*.

gynecology
The branch of medicine concerned with the diagnosis and treatment of disorders of the female reproductive system.

hallucination
A false sense of perception.

A hallucination can affect the senses of sight, hearing, taste, or smell; they range from something as simple as a flash of light to a detailed and clearly identifiable sight or sound.

Hallucinations may be symptomatic of a mental disorder or the result of physical illness. Recurring and often terrifying hallucinations may accompany high fever, alcoholism, drug abuse or severe injury. Disease or a tumor of the brain may cause hallucinations related to a particular sense depending on the area of the brain affected.

hay fever
An allergy to pollen manifested by cold–like symptoms; pollinosis.

Hay fever is a short–lived, seasonal, allergic reaction to the pollen of a particular plant or group of plants.

Common symptoms of hay fever include itchy watery eyes, sneezing, a watery discharge from the nose, headache, irritability, a feeling of tiredness, insomnia, coughing, and wheezing.

A number of over–the–counter remedies are available to the sufferer including antihistamines that counteract the histamine released by the body in reaction to the allergen, corticosteroids that reduce inflammation, and eye drops to relieve itching and redness. Severe cases may warrant consultation with a physician who can prescribe desensitization shots that induce the body to develop a tolerance to the allergen.

head

The upper part of the human body, housing the brain and organs for sight, hearing, smell and taste, joined to the trunk by the neck.

The head is composed of twenty–two bones, eight that are closely united to form the *skull*, a bony case that encloses and protects the brain; fourteen other bones form the face. The only movable joint in the head is the lower jaw.

hearing

The sense which allows us to receive and distinguish various sounds. Sound is basically made up of vibrations of varying magnitude, transmitted through a solid, a gas, or a liquid.

In the human body, the outer ear perceives or 'collects' sound waves or vibrations from the air and directs them through the ear canal to the eardrum. The vibrations of the eardrum travel through the middle ear where they are amplified and passed to the inner ear cochlea where tiny hairs are excited according to the magnitude of the vibrations. Finally, the auditory nerve picks up the signals from the hairs in the cochlea and passes them on to the brain where they are distinguished as sounds.

heart

The heart is a hollow, muscular organ about the size of a fist, lying in the lower central region of the chest cavity. By the heart's pumping action, blood is under pressure and in constant circulation throughout the

heart attack

body. In a healthy adult at rest, the heart contracts between sixty and eighty times a minute; in a child, eighty to a one hundred times per minute.

heart attack

A sudden diminishing of the heart's ability to function; myocardial infarction.

Like all living tissue, the muscles of the heart require oxygen–rich blood to function. A heart attack occurs when the blood supply to the heart is cut off by damage or blockage to the coronary artery that delivers blood to the heart muscle.

Diseases of the heart and blood vessels are the leading cause of death in the United States. Some of the early signs of a heart attack are uncomfortable pressure, squeezing, fullness, or dull pain in the center of the chest; pain radiating into the shoulders, arm, neck or jaw; sweating; nausea; dizziness; shortness of breath; or a feeling of weakness. The symptoms may come and go, leaving the impression that they are attributable to another cause such as indigestion.

Certain factors have been identified as increasing an individual's risk of some form of cardiovascular disease. There are some factors over which a person has no control, such as sex, race, age and heredity; however, there are factors that can be controlled, such as diet, weight, smoking, physical condition, etc.

heartburn

A burning sensation usually centered in the middle of the chest near the sternum. Heartburn is not normally associated directly with the heart, but is caused by the reflux, or bubbling up, of acidic stomach fluids so that they enter the lower end of the esophagus.

Because the reflux can increase the heart rate and heartburn does exhibit symptoms similar to angina, a physician should be consulted if symptoms persist or bouts of heartburn are frequent.

heart murmur

An abnormal heart sound that can usually be detected only with the aid of a stethoscope.

Generally, heart murmurs are harmless, but they can be early indicators of heart disease or a structural abnormality, such as a hole in the wall between the chambers of the heart, or incomplete closure or obstruction of a valve.

A heart murmur may be congenital, or the result of disease.

heat cramps

Severe cramps caused by severe loss of salt.

Heat cramps mostly affect those who work or play a hot environment and perspire profusely; the perspiration causes a loss of salt from the body and if there is inadequate replacement, the body will then suffer from cramps, often accompanied by a feeling of faintness.

The symptoms can usually be relieved by moving to a cooler area and drinking a commercial electrolyte solution or a teaspoon of salt and as much sugar as possible dissolved in a quart of water.

heat exhaustion

A condition caused by prolonged exposure to a hot environment.

heat stroke

Heat exhaustion occurs most commonly to persons not accustomed to hot weather, those who are overweight, and those who perspire excessively.

Loss of water and salt through sweating causes mild shock evidenced by pale and clammy skin, rapid and shallow breathing, rapid and weak pulse, nausea, weakness, dizziness, or headache.

One suffering from heat exhaustion should be moved to a cool, but not a cold place and wiped with cool, wet compresses on the face and head; if fainting seems likely, lie down with feet elevated eight to twelve inches.

heat stroke

A state of collapse brought on by exposure to heat; sunstroke.

Heat stroke is a sudden onset of illness from exposure to high temperature, often the direct rays of the sun. Physical exertion and high humidity contribute to the incidence of heat stroke.

The most dangerous characteristic of heat stroke is high body temperature caused by a disturbance in the heat regulating mechanism of the body. The sufferer can no longer sweat, and this causes a rise in body temperature. This illness is most common in the elderly, alcoholics, obese persons, and those on medication.

Symptoms exhibited by a victim of heat stroke are: skin that is flushed, very hot, and very dry; pulse that is strong and rapid, but may become weaker and rapid as the condition worsens; respiration that is rapid and deep, followed by shallow breathing; high temperature; a loss of consciousness and,

possibly, convulsions.
It is most important to lower body temperature as quickly as possible; failure to do so may result in permanent brain damage or death. In addition the subject should be: moved to a cool, but not cold, environment and all clothing removed; wrapped in a cool, moist sheet and fanned or immersed in cool water or wiped with cool compresses; transported to a medical facility as rapidly as possible, continuing cooling enroute.

hematemesis

Vomiting of blood.
Hematemesis may be caused by a simple irritation of the stomach, as by aspirin or overindulgence in alcohol, or it may be an indication of more serious illness, such as ulcers or cancer.

hematology

The study of blood, blood–forming organs, and related diseases.
Hematology is concerned with the diagnostic techniques for exploring disease processes through the examination of blood and bone marrow samples, as well as the workings, disorders and diseases of the blood and blood–forming organs themselves

hematoma

A swelling made up of blood, usually clotted; a bruise.
A hematoma is usually the direct result of trauma, although the blood may come from a vessel that is fragile or damaged by disease. Most hematomas heal without treatment, but there is a danger of infection, especially around the nose and eyes. Any unusual

behavior or complaint of headaches several days after an injury should be referred to a physician.

In cases of severe trauma, internal hematomas may develop. These too, will usually heal without treatment, although injuries to the head carry the possibility of belated symptoms of headache, drowsiness or paralysis that signal more serious injury that must be treated quickly.

hemodialysis See *dialysis*.

hemoglobin

The substance in red blood cells that enables them to carry oxygen and gives them their color.

hemophilia

A hereditary disease in which improper clotting of blood puts the sufferer in danger of a severe loss of blood from a minor cut or injury.

hemorrhage

The escape of blood from an artery, vein or capillary.

Hemorrhage often refers to considerable loss of blood, or uncontrolled bleeding. Normally, when blood vessels are torn or broken, the blood quickly forms clots, stemming the flow; however, when serious injury or disease, such as hemophilia, peptic ulcer, or cancer is involved, the body's normal clotting mechanism may malfunction or prove inadequate.

The seriousness of hemorrhage depends on the location and amount of bleeding. Severe hemorrhage may cause rapid pulse, dizziness, a drop in blood pressure, a rise in pulse rate, and clammy or sweaty skin. Blood in the stool, urine, or vomitus may be an indication of internal bleeding and should be reported to a physician as quickly as possible.

hepatitis

Inflammation of the liver.

Hepatitis usually refers to one of a number of viral infections, characterized by jaundice. The most common are hepatitis A or *infectious hepatitis* and hepatitis B or *serum hepatitis*, both of which attack cells in the liver.

Hepatitis A is transmitted through contaminated food, water or contact with the stool of an infected person. The infection may be so mild as to be without symptoms, although the infection can still be passed on to others.

Hepatitis B virus enters the bloodstream through contact with contaminated blood or other body fluids. The virus can exist in most body fluids, including blood, saliva, semen, urine, and tears; thus, it may be transmitted by sexual contact or, infrequently, by casual contact.

Hepatitis may cause fatigue, joint and muscle pain, loss of appetite, nausea, vomiting, and diarrhea or constipation, accompanied by a low grade fever. As the disease progresses, the liver may enlarge and become tender. The characteristic jaundice is caused by the accumulation of bile pigment in the blood that turns the skin and the whites of the eyes yellow.

The disappearance of jaundice generally signals the start of recovery from hepatitis A; the hepatitis B virus, however, may persist for years or even a lifetime.

Any suspicion of hepatitis infection requires medical

attention to avoid permanent liver damage. Although there is no cure, the physician can recommend a diet and life style that minimizes strain on the liver.

heredity

The transmission of characteristics from parent to offspring.

Each characteristic that may be transmitted is conveyed by a gene, the primary unit of heredity. Genes are arranged on chromosomes in a precise order and every human cell is comprised of forty–six chromosomes arranged in twenty–three pairs.

On inception, the two halves of the chromosomes that are to join split and reunite; thus one half of the new chromosome that will make up a unique new individual comes from each parent.

It is this pairing of chromosomes and the genes they carry that determine the characteristics of the offspring—basically, if the characteristic carried by the genes of both parents are the same, such as for color of eyes or hair, that characteristic will be carried by the offspring; if they are different, then the dominant trait is manifest, as for brown eyes over blue; however, the offspring will always carry the brown–blue pair of genes, so that such a person might mate with another person with a brown–blue pairing and the random splitting of the chromosomes can cause a blue–blue pairing in their offspring.

Other features that are inherited, as the tendency to develop certain diseases are not so clearly defined by a single gene.

hernia

The protrusion of a body part through a defect in the

wall that surrounds it.

A hernia may be congenital, or it may develop when muscle walls are weakened by strain or disease.

herniated disk

Protrusion of any of the disks that separate and cushion the vertebrae, or bones of the spinal column. The presence of a herniated disk usually becomes apparent only when the protuberance is large enough to press against a nerve and cause severe pain.

herpes

Any of a number of acute viral infections that are characterized by clusters of small blisters on the skin or mucous membrane.

Herpes simplex is a recurring form of herpes that usually affects the area around the mouth or the genitals. *Herpes zoster*, see **shingles**.

hiatal hernia

The protrusion of the stomach above the diaphragm; a hiatus or diaphragmatic hernia.

The diaphragm divides the chest cavity and the abdominal cavity. Normally, the esophagus passes through the diaphragm and connect to the stomach below. A hiatal hernia occurs when a portion of the stomach protrudes up into the chest cavity through the passageway used by the esophagus.

hiccup, hiccough

A sudden intake of air checked by closure of the glottis causing a sound typical to the condition.

The hiccup originates with irritation to a nerve that causes an involuntary spasm of the muscle of the diaphragm. The spasm causes a sharp intake of air that is stopped by the sudden closing of the glottis at the back of the throat. This sudden stop produces the characteristic jerk and sound.

The irritation to the phrenic nerve is usually caused by eating or drinking too fast. Unless an attack persists, the hiccup is of little significance.

Although cures for the hiccups abound, some rather bizarre, the most effective cure is holding the breath for as long as possible so as to suppress the response of the diaphragm.

hirsutism

Growth of hair that is excessive or that appears in unusual areas.

hives

An allergic condition characterized by itchy blotches or welts; urticaria.

Hives may be caused by allergens in food, as tomatoes, strawberries, etc.; certain drugs; bacteria; animal hair; or the environment, as exposure to cold or the sun.

An outbreak of hives may last less than an hour or continue for weeks, often subsiding, then reappearing from time to time. A mild attack is merely annoying, but more serious attacks may be accompanied by fever or nausea and even difficulty in breathing if the respiratory tract is infected. Treatment generally involves administering antihistamines.

Hodgkin's disease

A malignant disease of the lymphatic system; a type of lymphoma.

The cancer tends to attack lymph glands throughout

the body and often spreads to neighboring organs.

hookworm

A blood–sucking parasite that resides in the small intestine. The parasite usually gains entrance through the skin from contaminated soil and works its way into the small intestine. Its presence is detected by eggs in the stool.

Hookworms can cause harmful anemia in children.

hormone

A substance secreted by a gland and that is carried elsewhere to influence the function of specific cells or organs.

host

Any living thing, as a person, animal, plant, or organ, that offers a suitable environment to shelter a parasite, infection, etc.

Huntington's chorea, Huntington's disease

A rare hereditary degenerative disease of the central nervous system typified by progressive mental deterioration and involuntary movements.

hydrophobia See *rabies*.

hyperglycemia

An excess of sugar in the blood, as in *diabetes mellitus*.

hypertension

High blood pressure.

Blood flowing through the arteries at a pressure that is higher than normal places extra stress on the artery walls that can damage them and interfere with the blood supply to the heart, kidneys, and brain, causing heart attack, kidney failure, or stroke.

Hypertension exhibits no distinctive symptoms:

headache, fatigue, dizziness, ringing in the ears, frequent nosebleeds, etc. caused by high blood pressure are all symptoms that may be attributable to other causes.

To test for hypertension, a physician checks the blood pressure using a sphygmomanometer, a device with an inflatable cuff that is wrapped around the subject's arm and a gauge to indicate pressure.

Blood pressure is expressed as two readings: the *systolic* that is the pressure during a contraction of the heart; and the *diastolic* that is the pressure between beats. The cuff is inflated to stop the flow of blood through the artery and then gradually deflated so that with the use of a stethoscope, the physician can determine the pressure at which the first pulse is heard and, as the cuff continues to deflate, the pressure at which the stream of blood passing through the artery is heard. Normal adult pressure is about 120/80 although some variance from that standard is not abnormal. Both readings are of value to the physician in making a diagnosis.

Hypertension responds well to treatment; a minor variation from normal may require simply a change in lifestyle: weight loss, reduction of stress, a program of regular exercise, and a limitation of the intake of sodium. For more severe cases, medication may be prescribed.

hyperthyroidism

Any of the disorders that involve over activity of the thyroid gland.

The output of thyroid hormone is regulated by the thyroid gland's reaction to thyroid-stimulating hormone, produced in the pituitary gland when thyroid hormone is needed.

Hyperthyroidism occurs when the thyroid is no longer sensitive to this regulating mechanism, that is, thyroid hormone is produced even in the absence of thyroid–stimulating hormone.

Thyroid hormone is involved in a number of processes throughout the body, such as the regulation of body temperature, growth, fertility, and the conversion of food to energy. Such involvement portends a variety of symptoms, such as overheating, weight loss coupled with increased appetite, a reduction or cessation of menstruation, rapid heartbeat, hyperactivity and tremors.

Hyperthyroidism can be treated with a variety of medications, depending on the specific condition.

hyperventilation

Abnormally rapid or deep breathing, causing an excessive loss of carbon dioxide, that can make one light–headed or dizzy, or cause a loss of consciousness.

hypnosis

A passive state induced by suggestion.

A hypnotic state is brought about by having a subject in a quiet environment concentrate while a hypnotist quietly urges acceptance of the receptive state of mind.

Although not everyone can be hypnotized, and hypnotism is not often encountered in orthodox medicine, it has been successfully used in the suppression of pain certain symptoms, and the altering of harmful lifestyle patterns, such as smoking.

hypoallergenic

Descriptive of anything that is less likely than another similar product to cause an allergic reaction, often claimed of certain soaps and cosmetics.

hypochondria

Abnormal preoccupation with one's health.

Hypochondria may be a concern for health in general, imagining symptoms that change from time to time, usually after assurance by a physician that nothing is wrong, or obsession with a particular ailment or disease, or the condition of a specific organ.

hypoglycemia

An abnormal lack of sugar in the blood.

Normally, during digestion, insulin secreted by the pancreas reduces the level of blood sugar, called glucose, by enabling the body cells to absorb it.

Reactive hypoglycemia is triggered by the ingestion of food and occurs when too much insulin is secreted during digestion causing the cells over absorb it from the blood.

Fasting hypoglycemia is caused by inadequate conversion of carbohydrates into glucose, over absorption of glucose by the body, or an insulin producing tumor that does not respond to normal stimuli. At risk from fasting hypoglycemia are heavy drinkers whose sugar storage and release system in the liver is upset by alcohol or those who have not eaten for an extended period

Either type of hypoglycemia can cause fatigue, nervousness, inability to concentrate, dizziness, confusion, headache, hunger pangs, or visual impairment.

hypotension

Unusually low blood pressure.

Although high blood pressure can be a serious problem that leads to complications, in most cases low blood pressure is not threatening nor does it require treatment.

It is normal for blood pressure to vary, depending on factors such as age, sex, etc. Infrequently, a medical problem, such as certain types of heart disease, cause low blood pressure; in such cases, treatment of the condition corrects the hypotension.

One recurring symptom of hypotension may be that of dizziness when rising quickly from a sitting or reclining position. Normally, when such a move is made, the blood vessels contract to prevent a sudden loss of blood to the brain; however, for the sufferer of hypotension, this mechanism may not work properly, and he or she may find it necessary to rise slowly.

hypothalamus

A part of the brain that lies above the pituitary gland and regulates many body functions.

Through the pituitary gland, the hypothalamus affects the activities of the thyroid, pancreas, parathyroids, adrenals and sex glands. It is involved with the control of body temperature, sexual function, weight, fluid balance and blood pressure.

hypothermia

An abnormally low body temperature.

Hypothermia is a general cooling of the entire body— the inner core of the body is chilled, so that the body cannot generate heat to stay warm.

hypothyroidism

The condition usually occurs from immersion in cold water, but may be produced by exposure to extremely low air temperatures or to temperatures between thirty and fifty degrees Fahrenheit accompanied by wind and rain. Also contributing to hypothermia are fatigue, hunger, and poor physical condition.

Exposure begins when the body loses heat faster than it can be produced. When the body is chilled, it passes through several stages: the urge to move about and exercise in order to stay warm; shivering as an involuntary effort by the body to preserve normal temperature in the vital organs; deprivation of judgment and reasoning powers; feelings of apathy, listlessness, indifference, and sleepiness; a loss of muscle coordination. Cooling becomes more rapid as the internal body temperature is lowered; eventually hypothermia will cause coma and death.

hypothyroidism

A condition caused by under activity of the thyroid gland.

Thyroid hormone is involved in a number of processes throughout the body; see *hyperthyroidism*.

Hypothyroidism may be the result of a congenital defect, inflammation of the thyroid gland, or a deficiency of thyroid–stimulating hormone that causes insufficient production of thyroid hormone by the thyroid gland. Those with hypothyroidism tend to be overweight, easily tired, intolerant of cold, suffer dry hair and skin, etc.

hypoxia

A condition caused by a lack of oxygen in the body.

A lack of oxygen in the body may be caused by a lack of sufficient oxygen in the air breathed, as in mountain climbing or flying at high altitude; disease of the lungs that prevents oxygen from reaching the blood; or a reduction in blood circulating to the lungs due to heart failure or an obstruction of blood vessels in the lung.

hysteria
Any excessive emotional state.

A psychiatric condition in which one responds to anxiety or threat with uncontrolled emotional or physical reaction, as by extreme emotional outbursts, blindness, loss of speech, etc.

idiosyncrasy
That which is unusual in a person, as a mannerism, or reaction to a particular food.

ileostomy
A surgical procedure in which an opening is created in the wall of the abdomen and joined to an opening in the ileum, or lower part of the small intestine, to allow the elimination of body waste.

An ileostomy is created when the colon has been removed because of injury or disease, such as cancer.

Waste discharged through the opening is collected in a disposable bag that must be changed by the wearer. Once the diet is properly regulated, the ileostomy causes little restriction of normal activities.

immune response
The body's reaction to any invading organism.

Whenever the body is exposed to a foreign element,

an antibody is fashioned, specific to that element, and designed to surround and disable it. The immune response comprises the body's most effective defense against disease.

Once antibodies have been produced, they not only fend off the attack, but remain in the blood to protect against the next attack. So effective are these antibodies, that a second attack seldom occurs, that is, it is stopped before the infection can take hold, as in the case of chicken pox or measles virus where a single attack virtually guarantees immunity from a second attack for life.

This abiding presence of antibodies in the blood is the basis for immunization as well—the body is exposed to weakened or dead cells for which it forms antibodies that remain in the system. Some diseases require so—called booster shots, because the antibodies are known to lose their effectiveness after a time.

In some cases, antibodies are detrimental, as in the case of allergies, transplants and transfusions.

In the case of an allergic reaction, the immune system over reacts in the presence of a substance to which the body is especially sensitive, causing unpleasant symptoms, such as itching skin, runny nose, coughing and sneezing, or watery eyes.

An allergic reaction may be so mild as to go unnoticed, or it can be so severe as to be life threatening. Of particular concern is the severe reaction called *anaphylactic shock*, often caused by insect bites, that may cause difficulty in breathing. Each attack triggers a new response, so that subsequent attacks are usually worse than the previous one.

In the case of a transplant, that is, the deliberate introduction of foreign tissue into the body, there is an attempt to destroy the intruder, making it necessary to introduce drugs to suppress the immune system. Such drugs present the additional hazard of leaving the body open to infection by other organisms that are not beneficial.

Transfused blood must be of the same type as the recipient's blood so that the immune system will not attempt to destroy it.

immune system See *allergy and immunology*.

impetigo

A highly contagious eruptive infection of the skin, most common in children.

incontinence

Inability to control the passage of urine and stool, most often found in infants and the elderly.

Incontinence may be an indication of a more serious condition, such as an obstruction, infection, or other illness.

indigestion

Impaired digestion; dyspepsia.

Belching, stomach pains, a feeling that the stomach is over full, a sour taste, and even nausea, are all signs of indigestion, usually brought about by poor dietary habits. Ingesting fatty foods, rich foods, spicy foods, an excess of alcohol, or irregular meals all make one a prime candidate for dyspepsia.

Indigestion is quite common and seldom causes more than temporary discomfort; however, if it is chronic, that is, occurs regularly after meals or frequently causes sleep to be interrupted, it may be warning of a more serious condition, such as ulcers and should be referred to a physician for diagnosis.

infection

The presence of an organism, such as a bacterium or virus that can have a harmful effect on the body.

Indicating any organism that can cause disease.

The disease caused by such organism.

inflammation

Redness and swelling, accompanied by heat and pain.

Inflammation is the way that living tissue responds to infection—it is symptomatic of the body's protective mechanism at work.

influenza

A contagious viral infection of the upper respiratory tract.

Influenza is characterized by symptoms similar to a cold, often accompanied by a fever, chills, aching muscles, headache, and a feeling of general malaise.

The flu is unique in its ability to circumvent the immune system, that is, once a population has been infected, the structure of the virus changes so that existing antibodies are not effective in fighting the next attack.

Because influenza spreads so rapidly throughout a community, it has been surmised that the virus is transmitted by airborne particles from an infected person

Influenza is unpleasant, but seldom serious except for those with a condition that is aggravated by flu symptoms, as a respiratory infection or heart condition.

Treatment for the flu is basically the same as for a bad cold; bed rest, extra fluids, and aspirin or aspirin substitute to reduce fever and muscle aches.

An association has been established between administering aspirin for a viral infection and Reye's syndrome in children; therefore, aspirin should not be given to a child with influenza.

ingest

To take into the body by eating or absorbing.

inositol See *vitamin B complex*.

insect bites and stings

Although an insect bite or sting may be only a minor unpleasantness to most, those who have an allergic reaction to insect venom may suffer serious consequences.

An abnormal reaction to insect venom may be exhibited as swelling, tenderness and even a loss of feeling in the area of the bite that can be followed by shortness of breath, a rapid heartbeat, coughing, wheezing, and dizziness. In extreme cases, *anaphylactic shock,* a severe, potentially fatal, reaction can occur.

Unfortunately, as with most allergies, the reaction tends to grow more severe with subsequent attacks, so that one who has had a bad reaction would be prudent to avoid situations where the attack might be repeated, such as mowing the lawn, walking in the woods, etc.

Protection from severe allergic reaction may be accomplished with desensitization shots that help the body build up a tolerance. They comprise a series of shots with gradually increased doses of extract.

insomnia

The persistent inability to fall asleep or to remain asleep long enough to become rested. Insomnia is caused by a number of conditions. Sleep deprivation can be brought on by illness that causes discomfort or by a medication that makes it difficult for the brain to relax.

Probably the most common cause of insomnia is worry. One sleepless night leads to another so that even after the original problem is resolved, concern about not being able to sleep becomes the problem. In most cases, establishing a ritual before bedtime often helps—a short period of light exercise, employing a brief period of meditation or some other soothing technique, relaxing with a cup of herbal tea, etc. In extreme cases, sleeping pills may be necessary to return one to a normal sleep pattern, but they should be used with care because of the potential for dependence and the fact that they become less effective over time.

insulin

A hormone produced in the cells of the pancreas essential for body cells to absorb sugar.

Lack of an adequate insulin supply retards the absorption of sugar, causes it to build up in the bloodstream and leads to **diabetes mellitus**; an excess of insulin can cause over absorption by the cells and create a low level of sugar in the blood called **hypoglycemia**, that can lead to **insulin shock**.

insulin shock

An abnormal condition that occurs when there is an excess amount of insulin in the body.

Insulin aids in the absorption of sugar by the body cells. Too much insulin in relation to the amount of sugar available causes over absorption by the cells and a corresponding reduction of the level of sugar in the blood. When that level is too low, there is a reaction called *insulin shock*.

The prime causes of the condition are: not eating, so that not enough sugar has been taken in; taking too much insulin; or over exercising, thus burning sugar too fast.

The sufferer of insulin shock may experience a personality change, such as becoming confused or combative, headache, profuse perspiration, rapid weak pulse, dizziness, and cold, clammy skin. Eventually the condition leads to convulsions and unconsciousness.

One suffering from insulin shock requires immediate medical attention. Symptoms may be relieved temporarily by taking sugar in the form of orange juice, a candy bar, soft drinks, or several packets of sugar mixed with orange juice. The amount of sugar doesn't matter as the attending physician will balance the need for sugar against insulin production. It may be difficult to distinguish between a victim with insulin shock and one progressing into diabetic coma. When in doubt, administer sugar—giving sugar to a victim with too much blood sugar doesn't make any significant difference, but giving sugar to a victim in insulin shock can save a life.

internist

A physician who specializes in the diagnosis and nonsurgical treatment of disease.

intestines

The lower part of the alimentary canal, extending from the stomach to the anus; the large and small intestines.

iron deficiency anemia

An inadequate supply of iron in the body, usually caused by excessive bleeding. Most iron is stored in the blood, and an adequate supply is maintained from a normal diet that includes meat and dark green leafy vegetables, as well as that derived from red blood cells that break down within the body.

When a deficiency is suspected and there is no apparent reason for it such as menstruation or pregnancy, the assistance of a physician is required in order to find the underlying cause of the condition, such as internal bleeding from an ulcer.

ischemia

A deficiency of blood in an organ or part of the body. Ischemia is caused by obstruction of the blood vessels that supply an organ or area of the body. Such obstruction may be the result of narrowing, compression, or damage from conditions such as a blood clot or *atherosclerosis* and causes oxygen loss that leads to tissue death in the affected area.

jaundice

A condition caused by bile pigments in the blood, manifested by a yellowing of the skin and other tissue, and caused by disease or other abnormality. Often a disease causing the yellowing of the skin is itself called a jaundice.

joint

The juncture of two or more bones.

There are three types of joints: *immovable joints*, such as those in the skull; *joints with limited motion*, such as those of the ribs and lower spine, and *freely movable joints*, such as the knee, ankle, elbow, etc.
The bones are held in place by strong white bands, called ligaments, extending from one bone to another and entirely around the joint. A smooth membrane that lines the end of the cartilage and the inside of the ligaments secretes a fluid that keeps the joints lubricated.

kidney
One of a pair of abdominal organs that removes water and waste matter from the blood and excretes them as urine.

kidney dialysis See *dialysis*.

kidney failure
Descriptive of the condition that exists when the kidneys cease normal function, causing the buildup of toxic substances within the body.

Kidney failure may have any of numerous causes, such as: blockage of the urinary tract, as by kidney stones; an adverse reaction to medication; infectious disease that attacks the kidney; heart attack; severe dehydration; serious injury; or a congenital condition, one that exists from birth.

Kidney failure may be acute, when there is a sudden malfunction that causes a buildup of toxins within the body in a matter of hours, or it may be chronic, that is, a malfunction of the kidneys that grows progressively worse, with a gradual buildup of toxins, that may occur over a span of months or years.

The most common symptom of kidney failure is a

reduction in the output of urine that causes an accumulation of fluid in the tissues. As the body becomes more toxic, the subject experiences constant fatigue, loss of appetite, diarrhea, nausea and difficulty in breathing. If the condition remains untreated, coma and death will follow.

kidney stone

A mineral formation lodged in the urinary tract; a calculus.

Kidney stones are formed when excess minerals, such as calcium, are present and concentrate into a hard lump. They may exist without causing discomfort, or they may cause blockage that can interfere with normal function and cause considerable discomfort.

Excess calcium in the system may come from ingesting foods that have a high calcium content or those rich in vitamin D, that aids in the absorption of calcium, or from calcium released by fractured bones. Other factors may also contribute to the formation of kidney stones: uric acid may crystallize into stones; urine retained as the result of infection can contain a concentration of elements that can solidify.

When a stone becomes large enough, or becomes positioned so that it causes notice, it may cause considerable pain in the area, frequent and painful urination, blood in the urine, nausea, or chills and fever. A stone that becomes lodged in the ureter, the channel from the kidney to the bladder, can produce severe pain in the back, abdomen and groin. In any incidence of these symptoms, immediate medical attention is required.

Kidney stones that are too small to be noticed may still cause damage to delicate tissues in the urinary tract.

labyrinth

A complex of interconnecting anatomical cavities.

The inner ear.

labyrinthitis

An infection of the inner ear characterized by dizziness or vertigo that often causes nausea. Labyrinthitis is often caused by the spread of infection from an upper respiratory ailment such as cold or flu, but may be caused by bacteria as well. The best defense is prompt care by a physician when symptoms first appear.

laceration

A ragged cut or wound.

laryngitis

Inflammation of the larynx.

The larynx is the voice box located in the upper part of the respiratory tract. Infection of the larynx is manifested by a hoarse or grating voice, or occasionally, a complete loss of speech.

Laryngitis may be caused an infection, such as that accompanying a cold or flu, from irritation of the mucous membrane of the larynx, as by smoking, dust, or air pollution, or from straining the voice.

In addition to altered speech, the laryngitis sufferer may also experience a scratchy feeling in the throat and pain when speaking.

The best treatment for laryngitis is a total resting of the vocal cords and, if necessary, throat spray, aspirin, or acetaminophen to relieve discomfort.

Legionnaires' disease

Persistent or frequent recurrence may be sympto-matic of a more serious condition, and should be referred to a physician for diagnosis.

Legionnaires' disease

A severe bacterial infection of the respiratory tract.

The disease gets its name from what was thought to be its first outbreak—in 1976, among those attend-ing a convention of the American Legion in Philadel-phia. Subsequently, earlier outbreaks of the disease were identified, however.

Onset of the disease may be mild, emulating the on-set of influenza. Later symptoms are similar to those of any respiratory infection: coughing, shortness of breath, chest and abdominal pain, headache, fever, nausea, vomiting, and diarrhea.

Although outbreaks of the disease are infrequent, because of its life–threatening nature, it should be suspected in any respiratory infection that gets pro-gressively worse over a period of several days, espe-cially among the elderly or chronically ill.

leprosy

A mildly contagious, chronic bacterial infection that causes loss of sensation. If not treated, leprosy can cause paralysis, muscle atrophy, and deformity.

lesion

An alteration in the condition of tissue, that may be caused by injury, disease, abnormal growth, etc.

lethargy

An unnatural lack of energy; sluggishness.

leukemia

Any of a number of deadly diseases of the white blood cells and bone marrow.

Leukemia originates in the bone marrow, causing excessive production of white blood cells, many of which are immature or damaged. These ineffective white blood cells reduce the body's ability to fight infection while crowding out the red blood cells that carry oxygen throughout the body and platelets, that are necessary for clotting.

leukocyte

Any of the colorless cells found in the blood, lymph, or tissues, vital to the body's defense against disease or infection; a white blood cell.

ligament

Tough fibrous tissue that holds bones together at a joint and supports body organs.

lipoma

A benign tumor of fatty tissue.

lipoprotein

Any of a number of compounds in the body such as those formed by the combination of *cholesterol* with fats and proteins. Among the several types of lipoproteins in the body are LDL or low density lipoproteins that are associated with high blood pressure and heart disease, and HDL or high density lipoproteins that help to remove excess cholesterol from the blood and arteries.

liver

The largest gland in the body, located in the upper part of the abdominal cavity.

The liver performs a number of functions, including the manufacture of substances necessary for blood clotting, the processing of nutrients absorbed by the small intestine, and the removal of toxic substances from the blood.

living will

A document that specifies an individual's wishes regarding care and treatment if he or she becomes incapacitated, such as limiting life support that only prolongs dying. Most states have enacted laws regarding living wills, so it is important that the document be in accordance with the statutes of the state in which the subject resides.

lockjaw See *tetanus*.

lumbago

Rheumatic pain in the lower back; often used to describe any back pain.

Lyme disease

An infectious disease caused by a microorganism transmitted by ticks. The disease is characterized by a rash at the location of the bite and flu–like symptoms, such as fever, headache, and general malaise. Untreated, the disease can cause an arthritic condition, and attack the heart and nervous system as well. Ticks carrying the disease have been found mainly in the northeastern, upper midwestern, and northwestern parts of the U.S. Anyone who exhibits symptoms after a tick bite should consult a physician for, as with most infections, early treatment is the surest way to effect a quick cure.

lymphadenitis

A bacterial infection that causes painful inflammation of one or more lymph nodes. Because of the many conditions that can cause enlarged lymph nodes, such as cancer and cat–scratch fever, diagnosis requires the aid of a physician.

lymphocyte
A variety of white blood cell that develops in lymphatic tissue.
Lymphocytes are extremely important to the body's immune system—they identify the characteristics of *antigens*, produce the antibodies to combine with and destroy them, and direct immune responses.

lymphoma
Any of several cancers of lymphatic tissue, particularly of the lymph nodes.

malady
Any condition that exhibits symptoms of illness or disease.

malaise
A general feeling of discomfort or physical decline that may indicate the onset of disease.

malaria
An infection spread by the bite of a mosquito. The disease is characterized by high fever and profuse sweating often with a headache and a feeling of feebleness.
Malaria is mainly contracted in the tropics and there are preventive medicines available which vary according to the strain of malaria prominent in the area into which one is traveling. Treatment of the disease is effected by several drugs dependent on the type of malaria involved.

malignant
Descriptive of that which is a danger to health and well–being; likely to cause death.

malocclusion
Failure of the upper and lower teeth to meet properly

when the mouth is closed.
mastitis
An inflammation of the breast, especially of a nursing mother.
mastoid bone
The bone directly behind the ear.
mastoiditis
A bacterial infection of the air cells in the mastoid bone.

Mastoiditis is usually caused by the spread of infection from the middle ear. In severe cases, the infection is in danger of reaching the interior of the skull.

measles
A contagious viral disease common among children; rubeola.

The virus may be spread by moisture from the nose of throat of an infected person who is usually contagious for several days before symptoms are apparent and up to six days after the rash appears.

Early symptoms are similar to those of a cold—runny nose, congestion, sneezing, watery eyes, coughing and fever. After several days there is a sensitivity to bright light, the fever drops, and characteristic spots may appear in the mouth. Soon after, the fever rises and a rash appears, usually about the face, neck, and behind the ears before spreading over the entire body. The rash first appears as red spots; as they multiply, they grow together to form irregular blotches. Usually within days, the fever subsides and the condition improves. Although the disease is relatively mild, anyone contracting measles should be placed under a doctor's

care in order to avoid complications such as **pneumonia**, **encephalitis**, ear infection, **bronchitis**, etc.
As with all viral infections, aspirin should not be administered to children because of the link that has been established with Reye's syndrome.

melanoma
A tumor, usually malignant, of cells containing dark pigment.

Meniere's disease
A disorder of the inner ear caused by a buildup of fluid.

The canals, or labyrinth, of the inner ear serve to control balance and equilibrium by noting movements of the head and sending the information to the brain. Any disruption of this function can cause dizziness, nausea, vomiting, and distorted perception of surroundings, as when furniture appears to be spinning around a room.

Meniere's disease results from an increase in pressure from a buildup of fluid that distorts and, sometimes ruptures, the lining of the walls in the inner ear.

A mild attack may last less than an hour or several days, then disappear. Attacks may recur at intervals of weeks or months.

Severe attacks, that make normal movement impossible, require confinement to a bed. In the case of such attacks, bizarre illusions may accompany any head movement, the subject may suffer migraine headaches and some loss of hearing.

meningitis
An inflammation of the meninges, the membranes

that cover the brain and spinal cord that untreated can cause permanent disability or even death.

menses

The blood and cellular debris associated with an unfertilized egg that flows from the uterus when pregnancy does not occur after ovulation, approximately monthly during a female's reproductive years.

menstruation

The process of discharging the menses.

metabolic alkalosis See *alkalosis*.

middle ear infection

The middle ear serves to transfer sound vibrations to the inner ear and to protect the eardrum from rupture by equalizing the inside pressure with that on the outside of the body. Such equalization is made possible by the *eustachian tube* that connects the middle ear with the upper part of the throat.

The eustachian tube that protects the hearing is also the culprit that makes the middle ear susceptible to infection—most ailments of the middle ear are caused by virus or bacteria in the nose or throat that travel to the ear through the eustachian tube.

A middle ear infection can cause a severe throbbing pain, hearing loss, fever, dizziness, nausea, or vomiting. In extreme cases, the pressure against the eardrum may cause it to burst, relieving the pressure and attendant pain, but creating a danger of spreading the infection.

Because of the danger of hearing loss and spreading infection, a physician should be consulted in any case of ear infection.

mononucleosis

A contagious viral disease that attacks the lymph nodes; infectious mononucleosis.

Mononucleosis is characterized by a sore throat, fever, swollen glands, and a feeling of weakness. The onset of the infection is so subtle that it appears to be no more than a simple cold; however, a sore throat that persists for more than a week, with swollen glands in the throat and neck accompanied by fever and weakness may be a sign of mononucleosis.

The usual treatment for the condition is rest and lots of liquids until temperature returns to normal. As strength returns, a resumption of normal activity should have no ill effects.

Generally, mononucleosis is uncomplicated, although occasionally the infection spreads to the liver or spleen. Signs of its spread are *jaundice* and pain or tenderness in the abdomen. Either condition should be referred to a physician.

multiple sclerosis

A chronic disease of the nervous system.

The condition is the result of random destruction of the *myelin sheaths* that insulate nerve cells.

Multiple sclerosis usually affects young adults, causing weakness or paralysis in parts of the body, blurred vision, muscle spasms or incontinence. The disease then commonly goes into remission that may last several years, but recurring attacks can cause increasing disability.

For some, the condition does not become severe; for others, over time, extensive nerve damage causes a

mumps

loss of muscle control that precludes living a normal life.

mumps

A contagious viral disease most common among children.

An attack of mumps may begin with fever, headache, sore throat or earache followed by the characteristic painful swelling of the salivary glands that may cause difficulty in eating.

Other glands and organs may become infected and swollen as well, such as the testes, ovaries, pancreas, liver, etc.

muscle

Tissue made up of fibers that have the ability to contract.

It is through the contraction of muscle that all movements of the body are produced.

Voluntary muscles, also known as striated muscles are, with one notable exception, consciously controlled by the individual.

Involuntary muscles, also known as smooth muscles, such as those found in the blood vessels, digestive system, respiratory system, etc. are not under conscious control.

The exception to this ordering of muscles is a group of heart muscles that are striated, but controlled by the motor nerves rather than the conscious will.

myasthenia gravis

A neuromuscular disorder characterized by a slow and progressive paralysis.

Neuromuscular is a reference to nerves and muscular. Myasthenia gravis is a condition caused by a failure of muscles to receive messages transmitted by the nerves, causing paralysis, although the muscles do not atrophy, or waste away.

Signs of the disease usually show up first in the face as paralysis of the eye muscles that causes squinting or double vision, sagging of the cheeks, and difficulty in talking, chewing, or swallowing. The arms and legs may be affected, causing difficulty in walking or in the accomplishment of everyday tasks, like lifting a fork. Eventually, breathing may be impaired. The severity of symptoms varies from day to day and even throughout the day, with a tendency to be more oppressive at night.

There is usually no cure for myasthenia gravis, although there are drugs that can restore nerve transmission and improve muscle strength.

myocarditis

Inflammation of the myocardium, or muscle of the heart.

narcolepsy

A disorder characterized by sudden, uncontrolled lapses into deep, but brief, sleep.

Attacks may be related to another condition, although they often occur with no other symptoms: the subject simply falls into a deep sleep and awakens refreshed.

nausea

A feeling that one wants to vomit.

Nausea may be brought on by anything that interferes with the normal flow of nutriments through the digestive tract, whether direct, as in the case of reaction to tainted food or infection, or indirect, as by

necrosis

an emotional or psychological response.
Nausea may be manifested as discomfort or a burning sensation in the abdomen or chest, excessive secretion of saliva, sweating, blurred vision or feelings of weakness.

necrosis

Death of tissue in the midst of healthy tissue.
Necrosis takes place when cells are destroyed by infection or when they are cut off from their blood supply. It may occur in an area of the body served by vessels that have been injured or blocked, in areas of the heart following a heart attack, or in the midst of a tumor that has outgrown its blood supply.

neoplasm

Any abnormal growth of body cells or tissue; a tumor.

nephrology

The branch of medicine that deals with the diagnosis and treatment of kidney disorders.

nephrosis

A disease of the kidneys in which the filtration process permits protein molecules from the blood to be discharged in the urine. This depletion of proteins in the blood interferes with the passage of fluid from normal tissue and causes swelling throughout the body, particularly around the eyes, hands, and feet. When there are no other complications, the condition is not life threatening and is easily treated.

nervous system

The network of cells that receive and transmit signals to coordinate the various parts of the body and the organs controlling the body functions.

The main parts of the nervous system consist of the brain and spinal cord. The brain is a collection of nerve centers. Leaving the brain, the nerves join to the spinal cord, pass through the opening in the center of the backbone or spinal column and branch off to all parts and organs of the body.

There are mainly two types of nerves entering and leaving the spinal cord: sensory nerves that convey sensations such as heat, cold, pain, and touch from different parts of the body to the brain; and motor nerves that convey impulses from the brain to the muscles causing movement.

The nervous system consists of two separate systems by function: the voluntary and the involuntary. The *voluntary nervous system* is under control of the will, that is, movements and actions that are deliberate. The *involuntary nervous system* is a series of nerve centers in the chest and abdominal cavity along the spinal column. Each of these nerve centers is connected with the spine and the brain and controls vital organs and vital functions. This system is not under control of the will; through it involuntary muscles are stimulated to function without regard to the state of consciousness.

neuralgia

Descriptive of any pain along the course of a nerve.

The cause of neuralgia is not always apparent, although in some cases there may be evidence of inflammation or damage. The condition may be slight and fleeting, or it may involve a severe pain or one that is longer lasting.

Shingles, or *herpes zoster* is characterized by intense

pain and infection along the course of a nerve.

Sciatica, caused by pressure on the sciatic nerve, is experienced as an ache or a recurring tingling sensation in the buttock and along the back of the thigh.

Carpal tunnel syndrome causes tingling in the fingers that may progress to pain running up the arm as a result of pressure on the large nerve that passes through the wrist.

Treatment for these and other conditions that cause neuralgia varies with the cause, location and severity of the condition.

neuritis

Any inflammation of a nerve.

Neuritis may be brought on by infection, by pressure on the nerve, by exposure to toxins, by loss of the nerve's blood supply or by a lack of vital substances in the diet.

Neuritis can cause discomfort that ranges from tingling to severe pain, a loss of sensation and muscle control, or even paralysis.

Treatment for neuritis varies depending on the cause.

neurology

The branch of medicine concerned with the diagnosis and treatment of disorders that have an effect on the nervous system.

The nervous system comprises the brain, the spinal cord and the network of peripheral nerves that flows throughout the body.

neurosis

An emotional or psychological disorder.

Usually manifested by anxiety or depression, neurosis is commonly caused by the inability to adjust to the ordinary stresses of life.

neurotransmitter

A substance that transmits nerve impulses between nerve cells.

The basic unit of the nervous system is the nerve cell, or neuron. At the ends of each nerve cell are numerous sacs containing neurotransmitter chemicals that are released by nerve impulses traveling through the nerve cell. Upon their release, the neurotransmitters jump to the next nerve cell to stimulate the production of an impulse in that nerve cell to carry the signal on.

nosebleed

Bleeding from the nose caused by a rupture in the vessels in the inner lining of the nose.

Nosebleeds are usually caused by a blow to the nose, repeatedly blowing the nose, or long periods of breathing dry air. Occasionally they may be symptomatic of a more serious condition, as high blood pressure or a tumor.

Most nosebleeds can be stopped by leaning forward to avoid swallowing blood and pinching the soft portion of the nose for a few minutes, or by applying cold packs to the bridge of the nose.

Nosebleeds that are difficult to stop or recur regularly should be referred to a physician.

obesity

The condition of being significantly overweight.

obsession

That which engages a person's consciousness to an

abnormal degree.

Obsession may take the form of irrational concerns, repetitive actions, doubts, or fears that the subject cannot avoid or dismiss.

Obsessions may be linked, as in the case of one who repeatedly checks to see that the doors are locked because of an obsession with security.

An obsession may be a symptom of a psychiatric illness or of a brain disorder.

obstetrics/gynecology

Obstetrics is the branch of medicine that deals with conditions related to pregnancy and childbirth. *Gynecology* is concerned with the diagnosis and treatment of disorders of the female reproductive system.

Because of the close relationship between the two fields, they are often practiced as a single specialty.

occult blood

Blood in such small quantities that it cannot be easily detected.

Occult blood is usually descriptive of blood passed off in the feces that cannot be detected except under a microscope. Such blood is often a sign of bleeding in the gastrointestinal tract.

oliguria

An abnormal reduction in the passage of urine.

Oliguria may be a sign of kidney failure or other disease.

oncology

The study of the cause and treatment of abnormal tissue growth.

Oncology deals with tumors, particularly those that are malignant, or cancerous. Because of the close association with cancers of the blood, many oncologists are also hematologists, qualified to deal with diseases of the blood.

ophthalmology

The branch of medical science that deals with the study of the functions of the eye as well as the diagnoses, and treatment of diseases and injuries to the eye.

The ophthalmologist, who is a physician, may also qualify as a surgeon who can reattach retinas, remove cataracts, etc.

There are several non–medical fields that deal with the eyes, such as the *optometrist*, who tests the eyes for fitting out with corrective lenses, the *optician*, who fashions the lenses and fits glasses or contact lenses according to the prescription from the ophthalmologist or optometrist, and the *ocularist*, who fashions and fits artificial eyes.

ophthalmoplegia

Weakness or paralysis of the muscles of the eye.

Ophthalmoplegia affects the muscles that control eye movements as well as dilation and contraction of the pupil. It can be caused by any condition that impacts on the muscles or the nerves that control them, as a head injury, stroke, tumor, etc.

opiate

Any of a variety of sedative narcotics that are derived from the opium poppy (opium, morphine, or heroin), that contain opium, or that contain any of its synthetic derivatives.

opium

An addictive narcotic obtained from the juice of the

orthodontia

opium poppy
Opium is the source of morphine, heroin, codeine and other medicinal compounds.
Opium engenders a feeling of euphoria, relieves pain and hunger, and, in time, brings about drowsiness and sleep; however, the addictive nature of opium is so strong that most users become physically and emotionally dependent on the drug.

orthodontia
The branch of dentistry that deals with the correcting of irregularities of the teeth.

orthopedics
The branch of medicine that deals with disease and injury of the muscles, bones, and joints.

ossification
The transformation of soft tissue into bone or bone–like tissue.

osteoarthritis
A degenerative disease of the joints.
Osteoarthritis is generally associated with age, and is most prevalent in joints weakened by a prior injury or disease, or those subjected to unusual stress, as lower body weight–bearing joints, especially among the overweight.
The condition is caused by loss of the cartilage that normally protects the ends of the bones: as the space between the bones narrows, they may grate to cause wear or displacement of the bone and ultimately, inflammation, swelling, pain, and stiffness in the joint.

osteoma
A benign tumor comprised of bone.

An osteoma is seldom troublesome unless it is positioned to cause pressure on a nerve. The growth may appear anywhere in the body, but is most often attached to a normal bone, especially of the skull and the lower jaw.

osteomalacia

Softening of the bones.

Osteomalacia is caused by a lack of vitamin D, that is necessary for the absorption and utilization of calcium in the body.

Vitamin D is formed in the skin from exposure to sunlight and is available in the diet in dairy products, many of which are fortified with vitamin D, and in fish oils, that are rich in vitamin D. In some areas, a lack of winter sunlight to aid in the formation of vitamin D contributes greatly to the deficiency; however, regular doses of cod liver oil, available in capsules, can overcome the problem.

The deficiency of vitamin D may also be caused by any condition that inhibits its absorption even though it is present, or by an increased requirement for the vitamin, as in pregnancy.

Osteomalacia causes pain and tenderness in the bones, and may lead to bone fractures and weakness of the muscles.

osteoporosis

A condition marked by a decrease in calcium content of the bones.

As the body ages, the bones thin to some extent; when there is an abnormal lack of calcium available to the body, the process is hastened and the bones become especially susceptible to fracture.

osteosarcoma

The onset of osteoporosis may escape notice, or it may cause pain in the lower back, often following the fracture of a vertebra. Such fractures tend to be patterned, so that over a period of time, subsequent fracturing of vertebrae may lead to deformity of the spine and difficulty walking that can make one susceptible to further injury. Osteoporosis is a leading factor in the numerous hip injuries among the elderly.

The best defense is a carefully monitored program of light exercise that strengthens the muscles supporting bones that have become weakened by the disease. Diet is also any important factor, especially one that provides adequate vitamin D and calcium to promote the formation of bone.

osteosarcoma

A malignant tumor of the bone.

Osteosarcoma may infect any bone but usually occurs in the long bones of the arm or leg. Most common in children and young adults, the malignancy typically spreads to the lungs which is usually fatal.

otorhinolaryngology

The medical specialty that combines the study, diagnosis and treatment for diseases of the ears, nose and throat.

Because of the linkage of the passages between the ears, nose and throat—the ears and throat are linked by the eustachian tubes; the nose and throat meet at the nasopharynx—infections in one organ are commonly spread to another or to all.

otosclerosis

A growth of spongy bone in the ear that causes

progressive deafness.

In otosclerosis, the stapes, one of the bones in the middle ear that transmits sound waves to the inner ear, is overgrown and immobilized, so that the transmission of sound vibrations is impaired.

The condition may be corrected by a surgical procedure in which the stapes is replaced—a very delicate procedure that carries some risk of failure.

oxygen

A colorless, odorless gas that occurs free in the atmosphere.

Oxygen, essential to the body, is absorbed from the lungs into the bloodstream, where it is carried by the hemoglobin in the red blood cells to be discharged to the tissues.

The brain is most sensitive to organ deprivation and is permanently damaged if its supply is cut off for more than a few minutes.

pacemaker

A network of muscle fibers in the right ventricle of the heart that control the rhythm of the heartbeat; an artificial device that stimulates heart action and regularizes the heartbeat by the periodic discharge of electrical impulses.

It is the function of the natural pacemaker in the heart to cause it to beat at a regular tempo that allows for the proper flow of blood through it. When that natural function is impaired by injury or disease, an artificial pacemaker may be implanted in the heart to take over the function.

pain

Severe discomfort that may be physical, as that

caused by disease or injury, or emotional, as that caused by grief or depression.

The mechanics of pain are not thoroughly understood, but it is pain that assists greatly in the diagnosis of disease or injury as by location, type, or duration of the pain.

Paget's disease

A disease in which the body cells that are charged with the replacement of old bone cease to function in an orderly manner and produce enlarged, weakened bone structures. The disease is mainly one suffered by the aging and the condition often causes fractures and deformation. Mild forms of the disease may not be troublesome. Treatment of severe forms by a physician will vary depending on which bones are involved.

palate

The roof of the mouth, that consists of a firm *hard palate* in the front and a fleshy *soft palate* in the back, toward the throat.

palliative

Descriptive of medication that alleviates pain or other symptoms, but does not have the power to heal.

palpitation

Rapid beating, especially of the heart.

palsy

Any of a number of diseases characterized by tremors, weakness of the muscles, or an odd gait and attitude; paralysis.

pancreas

A large gland located near the stomach at the back

of the abdominal cavity that secretes enzymes to aid in digestion and hormones to regulate the level of sugar in the blood.

Enzymes produced by the pancreas are released to the small intestine to help break down carbohydrates, proteins and fats.

Hormones produced in the pancreas include insulin, that aids body cells in the utilization of glucose, or blood sugar, and glucagon, that prompts the liver to release stored sugar into the blood.

pancreatitis

Inflammation of the pancreas. The condition is characterized by a number of symptoms including abdominal pain, nausea, fever, accelerated heartbeat, and clammy skin. As there are a variety of causes for pancreatitis as well as treatment that varies with the cause, a physician must be consulted for a specific diagnosis.

paralysis

Impairment or loss of muscle function.

Paralysis may be caused by disease or injury to the muscle itself or to the part of the nervous system that directs it and may range in severity from impairing a single muscle or nerve to affecting a large part of the body.

Disease of the muscle itself commonly leads to weakness, rather than total paralysis, although in certain forms of *muscular dystrophy*, the disease can cause severe and ultimately fatal paralysis.

Any blockage of impulses from the nerves to the muscles, whether caused by direct injury or by disease may cause either weakness or lead to total paralysis, depending on the condition. Recovery, too, depends on the underlying cause, as in some situations there is total remission while in others there is virtually no hope for recovery.

paranoia

A mental disorder characterized by delusions of persecution and grandeur.

Paranoia is characterized by suspicions that otherwise innocent acts are direct personal attacks, coupled with an exaggerated feeling of self worth that the subject feels is unrecognized or unjustly ignored by others.

paraplegia

Paralysis of the lower part of the body.

Paraplegia, usually caused by damage to the spinal cord, may affect only the use of the lower limbs, or it may encompass the lower trunk as well causing dysfunction of the bladder and rectum.

parasites

A plant or animal that lives in or on another from which it gains sustenance or protection without returning any benefit, and perhaps doing harm to its host.

Parkinson's disease

A nervous disorder characterized primarily by tremor, muscle rigidity and a jerky gait.

The condition may be marked by uncontrollable shaking, difficulty in starting to move, a stooped posture and expressionless face. Shaking may be more noticeable with tension or excitement, or when resting. In the later stages, speech, eating and writing become more difficult.

Parkinson's disease is progressive; it may be present in a mild form for years with little change, or it can lead to severe disability within a few years.

pasteurization

The process of heating a liquid to maintain a temperature of 60° to 70°C. for about forty minutes.

Pasteurization destroys organisms that cause fermentation, thus retarding spoilage of the liquid, as well as those that cause disease in humans, such as the bacteria that causes tuberculosis.

patch test

A test to determine sensitivity to specific irritants.

Allergy, or excessive sensitivity to a substance such as pollen, feathers, or dust, or a chemical, such as a detergent, cosmetic or drug, is the cause of hay fever and hives, and may be the cause of many cases of asthma, eczema and sinusitis.

When the cause of an allergic reaction is not apparent, a patch test may be used to determine the irritant or irritants that are causing the reaction. The patch test is administered by applying a small patch of an irritant to the skin and checking for a reaction in one to two days. Because of the large number of possibilities, several irritants are usually tested at one time. Testing continues with different sets until it is determined which irritants cause a reaction, and treatment can begin.

pathology

The branch of medical science that deals with the nature of diseases.

Pathology is concerned with determination of the causes, symptoms and effects of disease as well as the means by which the spread of a disease may be limited.

There are a number of specialties within that of pathology. Best known, perhaps, is forensic pathology, which is charged with the gathering of information, as from an autopsy, to be used as evidence in a court of law.

pediatrics

The branch of medical science that deals with the diseases and care of children.

pellagra

A disease caused by a deficiency of niacin.

Niacin is a part of the complex of B vitamins, present in meat, eggs, vegetables and fruit.

Signs of pellagra are reddening of exposed skin, loss of appetite, and irritability. The condition is common among alcoholics.

pelvis

The pelvis is a basin–shaped bony structure at the lower portion of the *trunk*. The pelvis is below the movable *vertebrae* of the *spinal column*, which it supports, and above the lower limbs, upon which it rests.

Four bones compose the pelvis: the two bones of the backbone and the wing–shaped hip bones on either side. The pelvis forms the floor of the *abdominal cavity* and provides deep sockets in which the heads of the thigh bones fit.

peptic ulcer

Descriptive of any erosion, or open sore, in the area of the digestive tract exposed to pepsin.

Pepsin is an enzyme formed in the stomach that aids

in the digestion of proteins. Although unconfirmed, it is believed that peptic ulcers are the result of excessive excretions of pepsin irritating the walls of the lower end of the esophagus, the stomach, or the duodenum, the first portion of the small intestine. Natural weakness in the wall of the stomach may also contribute to the problem, as does stress and heredity.

The onset of ulcers may be subtle, exhibiting symptoms that can be taken for indigestion; however, when the symptoms appear after every meal, during stress, and occasionally, just before meals, a physician should be consulted.

pericarditis

Inflammation of the pericardium, the membrane that surrounds the heart.

Pericarditis may be associated with other infections or diseases, such as pneumonia or a heart attack, or it may be caused by bacteria that enters the body through an open wound.

The condition is marked by chest pains that intensify with breathing, coughing or lying down. Other illnesses with similar symptoms are equally serious; therefore, any incident of chest pain should be referred to a physician.

A condition called *constrictive pericarditis* occurs when inflammation causes thickening of the pericardium that restricts heart action. The condition is marked by difficulty breathing, swollen neck veins and accumulation of fluid in the legs.

periodontics

The branch of dentistry that deals with the study

peritonitis

and treatment of diseases and disorders of the periodontium, that is, the gum and tissues surrounding and supporting the teeth.

peritonitis

Inflammation of the peritoneum, the membrane that lines the abdominal cavity.

Peritonitis can be caused by perforation of one of the hollow organs of the abdomen, an infection spread from an inflamed organ, or breaching of the abdominal cavity by a wound from the outside.

The condition is characterized by intense pain and the abdominal wall becomes tender and rigid. There may be nausea, vomiting; and dehydration. Peritonitis is extremely serious and requires immediate medical attention.

pertussis See *whooping cough*.

phantom limb syndrome

The illusion by an amputee that the missing limb is still in place.

The individual may experience feelings of touch, heat, cold, pain, etc. Usually the sensations disappear as the subject recuperates, but they may last for a considerable time or reappear without notice, especially feelings of pain.

pharmaceutics, pharmacy

The craft of the precise preparation and dispensing of medicines according to the instructions of a licensed physician.

In addition, the pharmacist has the knowledge to advise on the use of non–prescription medications.

pharmacology

The study and acquired knowledge of the nature and

action of drugs.

pharyngitis

Inflammation of the pharynx, the passage that connects the back of the mouth and nose with the larynx and esophagus; sore throat.

phlebitis

Painful inflammation of a vein evidenced by swelling and sensitivity in the area of the inflammation.

pituitary gland

A tiny organ located just beneath the base of the brain that produces a number of hormones that direct the functions of other glands and organs throughout the body.

platelets

Disk–shaped structures in the blood that play a critical part in clotting; thrombocytes.

Normally, the lining of a blood vessel allows the blood to flow without change in its chemistry; however, when a blood vessel is ruptured and the blood comes into contact with foreign tissue, clotting begins. *Platelets* in the blood, triggered by the contact, release a chemical that begins a chain reaction involving a number of protein constituents in the blood, ending with the conversion of fibrinogen, a soluble material, to fibrin, that is insoluble. The fibrin is laid down in fine strands that collect white and red blood cells to form a clot.

pleurisy

Inflammation of the pleura, the membranes that cover the outer surface of the lungs and the inner surface of the chest cavity.

The pleurae, lubricated by pleural fluid, serve to

reduce the friction of chest members moving against one another as the lungs expand and contract.

Pleurisy frequently occurs as a secondary complication of a respiratory tract infection, such as pneumonia, though there are other causes.

Dry pleurisy describes the condition where the infected pleurae rub against each other; *wet pleurisy* is characterized by a condition in which fluid from the infected tissue fills the space between the pleurae or, effectively, between the lungs and the wall of the chest cavity. In either case, breathing is painful and difficult. Breathing capacity may be especially reduced in the case of wet pleurisy because the fluid in the chest cavity tends to compress the lungs.

In addition to severe chest pains that force shallow breathing, there is usually fever and a painful cough.

pneumonia

Inflammation of the lungs, in which the air sacs in the lungs, the alveoli, fill with fluid and white blood cells.

Pneumonia is classified primarily according to the location of the inflammation: *lobar pneumonia* is a type of pneumonia that is usually confined to one section, or lobe, of the lung; *double pneumonia* is a condition that affects both lungs; *bronchial pneumonia* is concentrated in and about the bronchi, the airways that connect the windpipe and the air cells of the lungs; *walking pneumonia* is descriptive of a relatively mild condition that may not be readily identified as a lung infection.

Pneumonia may be caused by bacteria, virus, fungi

or other microorganisms. Any foreign matter, such as a chemical, food or vomit, that is inhaled may carry an agent that causes infection. Any type of drug or disease that inhibits the immune system may make one increasingly susceptible to an attack of pneumonia.

Pneumonia commonly occurs when resistance is lowered, as by another infection, or a disease that affects the entire body. It may be brought on when the body's defenses are strained from fighting the ravages of a cold, influenza, emphysema, asthma, etc.

Any condition that requires confinement to bed for a long period increases susceptibility to pneumonia, especially in the elderly.

Pneumonia is usually characterized by chest pain, fever, coughing, and difficulty in breathing. Pneumonia caused by a viral infection may be preceded and accompanied by the symptoms normally associated the a cold or flu. Other forms of pneumonia may strike suddenly with chills, shivering, an abrupt rise in temperature, shallow breathing, and the discharge of dark yellow or bloody sputum.

General treatment for pneumonia should be with the advice of a physician, and usually involves bed rest, plenty of fluids and a soft diet. If the condition is secondary to another, treatment of the primary condition is important in order to strengthen the body's immune system. Bacterial pneumonia may be treated with antibiotics.

In very serious cases, or where there is continued labored breathing, hospital care may be necessary.

podiatry
The science that deals with diseases, irregularities and injuries of the foot; chiropody.
Not all problems of the feet require a specialist, but some, such as correction of a deformity occurring at birth, should be in the hands of one likely to be most knowledgeable about the latest techniques.
The podiatrist often fills a special need by performing normal foot care that the elderly or incapacitated cannot perform for themselves, and by the knowledge and treatment of those conditions that most effect the elderly.

poisoning
The introduction into the body of any substance in a quantity that is harmful or destructive.
Poisoning may be deliberate or it may be accidental. It may be caused by an otherwise non–toxic or even beneficial substance, as a medication in combination with another substance, or in a large quantity or *overdose*, that makes it harmful. It may come in the form a pollutant in the air or a bacterial growth in tainted food.
Poisoning can produce unpleasant symptoms, such as abdominal cramps, nausea, vomiting, sweating, or a feeling of weakness. It can also cause delirium, loss of consciousness, difficulty in breathing, blindness, paralysis and death.
Certain poisons may be neutralized or passed off by the body while others, ingested in small quantities accumulate in the system until they become damaging. Some cases of poisoning have no lasting effect while others cause scarring or other conditions that

remain and may get worse in time.

Treatment for poisoning may be as simple as cleansing the offending substance from the body or administering an antidote, or it may require extended treatment to correct the resulting damage.

poliomyelitis

An inflammation of the spinal cord that can cause paralysis; infantile paralysis; polio.

Poliomyelitis is a viral infection, spread by inhalation or ingestion of dust or fecal matter, that can reach epidemic proportions.

Infection initially causes discomfort or cramps in the muscles, sore throat, and a stiffness in the neck and spine. Symptoms may recede within a few days or they may spread throughout the system, causing paralysis, atrophy of the muscles and, in some cases, permanent disability.

Immunization is so widespread that it has been practically eradicated in the United States.

polyp

A projecting growth of mucous membrane, usually not malignant.

proctology

The branch of medical science that deals with diseases and disorders of the anus and rectum.

prognosis

A prediction of the probable course of a disease or disability and the forecast for recovery.

prosthesis

An artificial device that replaces a natural part of the body.

The most common prosthetic device is one that

replaces missing teeth: dentures, false teeth, partial plates, etc.

Other prosthetic devices include artificial limbs; replacement joints, such as for the hip, knee, elbow, etc.; replacement valves for the heart; and replacement lenses for the eye. Some devices are strictly cosmetic, such as an artificial eye that has no function except to replace an eye lost to disease or injury.

proteinuria

The presence of protein in the urine. ***Albuminuria*** is virtually the same as proteinuria, since albumin is the only protein detected in significant amounts in the urine.

psoriasis

A chronic skin disease characterized by reddish patches of skin with silvery scales.

Psoriasis is not contagious.

psychiatry

The branch of medicine dealing with the diagnosis and treatment of mental and emotional diseases and disorders.

The *psychiatrist* is a medical doctor with training in psychology and is therefore authorized to prescribe medication as a part of therapy; the *psychologist*, on the other hand, does not have a medical degree and thus cannot prescribe drugs.

In addition to the treatment of *psychoses*, that is, severe mental disorders, psychiatry is involved in the treatment and rehabilitation of those suffering from behavioral disorders, anxiety, depression, addiction, etc.

psychology
The science that deals with human behavior; the study of mental and emotional processes.

psychosis
A severe personality disorder in which contact with reality is seriously impaired.

Psychosis may be the result of malfunction of the mind without apparent organic cause, or it may be caused by injury or disease.

psychosomatic
Descriptive of a physical ailment that originates in a mental or emotional disorder.

pulmonary medicine
The branch of medicine that deals with the study, diagnosis, and treatment of diseases and disorders of the lungs.

Pulmonary medicine is concerned with the care and treatment of such diseases as cancer of the lungs, tuberculosis, pneumonia, bronchitis, pleurisy, and emphysema.

purpura
The presence of blood in the skin or mucous membranes.

Purpura is caused by defects in the walls of capillaries that have not been sealed off by platelets.

The condition is evidenced by tiny red or purple spots appearing on the surface of the skin or mucous membrane.

pus
A yellowish–white fluid in which dead leukocytes, dead tissue, etc. are suspended; the result of an infection.

pustule
A small eruption on the skin filled with pus.

quarantine
The isolation of those who have been exposed to a communicable disease.

The purpose of a quarantine is to limit exposure to a dangerous, communicable disease so as to prevent its spread to others, especially when there is danger of an epidemic, or rapid spread throughout the community.

Quarantine is not necessarily limited to those who show signs of being infected. Once there is exposure to certain diseases, an individual who is susceptible may be infected and not show symptoms for a time, although the disease can be passed on to another. That period of incubation varies depending on the disease. By isolating the person or persons for the longest known incubation time of the disease, there is reasonable assurance that the infection has not been passed on.

rabies
An infectious, fatal, viral disease of animals that can be transmitted to man.

The rabies virus is contained in the animal's saliva; humans usually contract the disease from the bite of an infected animal.

Early symptoms of the disease are depression, restlessness and fever followed by a period of hyperactivity, abnormal salivation and painful spasms of the muscles in the throat. Usually, the victim develops an aversion to water, being unable to drink despite an irrepressible thirst. An untreated case is usually fatal in three to ten days.

To avoid rabies infection, treatment of any possible exposure should be prompt. After a bite, or any exposure of an open wound to animal saliva, the area should be completely washed with soap and water, and swabbed with an antiseptic, then seek medical help.

A domestic animal that does not exhibit symptoms should be confined and observed. A wild animal or any animal that shows symptoms of being rabid should only be captured by an experienced professional.

radiation therapy

The treatment of disease by the use of radioactive materials.

Such treatment may be by material contained in a device that can be inserted directly into the tissues or a body cavity, or in an injection, or as a drink.

radiology

The branch of medicine that treats of the use of radioactive substances in the diagnosis and treatment of disease.

Diagnostic radiology is mainly involved with the use of X rays to reproduce an images of part of the body on X–ray film. To improve the quality of the image and the subsequent analysis, special dyes called *contrast media* may be used in certain circumstances. Radiologists also use sound waves or magnetic impulses to create images.

Radiation oncology is a special field concerned with the application of radiation as a treatment for cancer.

rash
> A skin eruption, usually red spots or patches, often with minor irritation, as itching.
> A rash may be symptomatic of a number of conditions, including blocked sweat glands, allergy, viral or bacterial infection, etc.

reflex
> An automatic, involuntary, or learned response to a stimulus.
> Most of the actions of the body that allow it to function normally are reflex actions, such as the release of perspiration to adjust body heat, the secretion of digestive juices when food is ingested, or the adjustment of the eye to accommodate available light.
> Many such reflexes are conscious, or controllable; for example, the reflex that closes the eye when an object is brought near may be overcome to allow examination by a physician.
> Many reflexes are learned as well: experience often dictates whether one ducks or tries to catch a thrown object.
> The failure of the body to respond in a normal or expected way to stimuli may also be a sign of disruption in the neural function.

respiration
> Inhaling and exhaling; the exchange of oxygen and carbon dioxide between the outside air and the lungs.

respiratory alkalosis See *alkalosis*.

respiratory arrest
> A cessation of breathing.
> Breathing may stop as a result of a variety of serious

accidents. The most common causes of respiratory arrest are overdose of narcotics; electric shock, which can cause paralysis of the nerve centers that control breathing and stop or alter the regular beat of the heart; suffocation or drowning, a form of suffocation, in which air to the lungs is cut off by water or spasms of the larynx; poisonous gas, such as carbon monoxide, sulfur dioxide, oxides of nitrogen, ammonia, or hydrogen cyanide; head injuries, and heart problems.

respiratory system

The system by which oxygen is taken into the body and carbon dioxide is discharged, comprising the nose, throat, larynx, trachea, bronchi and lungs.

Oxygen enters the body through *respiration*, the breathing process.

During respiration, air is taken into the lungs and forced out the air passes through the nose, throat, and windpipe.

The throat is a continuation of the nose and mouth. At its lower end are two openings, one in front of the other: the opening in front, the trachea or windpipe, leads to the lungs.

As the windpipe extends into the chest cavity toward the lungs, it divides into the two bronchial tubes, one going to each lung. The lungs are two cone-shaped bodies that are soft, spongy, and elastic.

During breathing, the chest muscles and diaphragm expand the chest cavity, so that the air pressure within the chest cavity becomes less than that outside. Air rushes in to balance the pressure, filling the lungs.

During inhalation the ribs are raised and the arch of the diaphragm falls and flattens, increasing the capacity of the chest cavity, and causing air to enter. In exhalation, an act normally performed with slight muscular action, the ribs fall to their normal position, the arch of the diaphragm rises, decreasing the capacity of the chest cavity, and air is forced out.

At rest, a healthy adult breathes about fifteen times a minute and takes in twenty–five to thirty cubic inches of air per breath. Each breath moves about one–half liter (500 cc, or one pint) of air. During strenuous work, the breathing rate and amount inhaled may increase several times.

retina

The light–sensitive organ at the back of the eye that receives images from the lens that are transmitted through the optic nerve to the brain.

Reye's syndrome

A serious disease in which inflammation of the brain is coupled with liver damage.

Reye's syndrome is a rare condition that usually infects children recovering from a viral infection, such as chicken pox. A relationship has been established between contraction of the disease and the administering of aspirin for a viral infection, therefore, it has been advised that aspirin not be given to children recovering from chickenpox or any similar malady. No exact cause for the disease is known.

The onset of the infection is characterized by sudden vomiting, hyperactivity or sleepiness, and confusion. Convulsions and coma may follow.

Immediate diagnosis is essential as the first few days

of the disease are usually the most critical.

rheumatic fever

An infectious disease characterized by swelling of the joints and inflammation of heart valves.

Rheumatic fever, most common in children, is brought about by an allergic reaction following a bacterial infection of the throat.

The condition is evidenced by painful inflammation and swelling as the joints of the ankles, knees, and wrists are infected one by one; the development of large, irregular skin rashes; and fever. Inflammation of the valves of the heart may cause permanent damage due to the formation of scar tissue that prevents the valves from opening and closing properly. Problems of the heart may surface years after the initial infection when the overworked heart becomes enlarged.

Any time a throat infection is followed within a few weeks by fever and inflammation of the joints, rheumatic fever should be considered, and a physician should be consulted.

rheumatic heart disease

A complication of an attack of *rheumatic fever*.

Rheumatic fever, as noted above, may cause inflammation of the heart valves that results in the formation of scar tissue. The valves thus damaged may function without symptoms of impairment for years or even decades.

Heart murmur is a common symptom caused by blood flowing past a damaged valve. Although it is possible for the heart to compensate for the damage so that there is no serious disability, significant problems may occur. The scarring can cause a narrowing of the valve that restricts the flow of blood. Blood clots may form to further restrict the flow of blood out of the heart and lead to a number of symptoms associated with the deprivation of oxygen in the organs of the body.

Under the care of a physician, a program of regular exercise and proper diet can, in most cases, minimize the effects of rheumatic heart disease.

rheumatology

The branch of medicine that deals with the study, diagnosis, and treatment of rheumatic diseases, that is, those concerned with connective tissue, as bones and muscles.

Rh factor

A specific antigen that is present in some blood.

An antigen is a potentially harmful substance in the body that starts the reaction leading the body to produce a special *antibody* to neutralize it. Antigens commonly are introduced into the body by invading bacteria or other infecting agents.

The Rh, or rhesus, factor, named for the monkey in which it was first discovered, is found in certain blood, designated *Rh–positive*. *Rh–negative* blood is that blood lacking the Rh factor.

If Rh–positive blood is introduced into the bloodstream of one who has Rh–negative blood, antibodies are produced, because the Rh–negative immune system is unfamiliar with the Rh factor and views it as an invader.

Mixing of the different bloods can come about in two ways: by the transfusion of Rh–positive blood to an

Rh–negative person, or through the mixing of the blood of an Rh–negative mother with that of a child who has inherited Rh–positive blood from the father. In either case, the Rh factor in the Rh–positive blood will cause the Rh–negative system to form antibodies to trap and destroy the offending Rh factor. Such action causes the formation of clumps in the blood that can create a stoppage that will result in death.

As with all allergies, the first exposure may not cause a serious reaction because of the time required for the body to form anti–bodies. The second transfusion or pregnancy, however, when the antibodies are already present in the blood and the immune system is ready to produce more, will almost always cause severe complications.

Careful typing of blood and the development of a substance that disables the Rh antibodies have made complications from Rh incompatibility relatively rare.

rickets

A deficiency disease of children that often causes bone deformity.

Those who contract rickets tend to exhibit swollen joints or distortion of limbs and other deformities caused by softened and irregular bone growth that is the result of insufficient vitamin D to aid in the absorption of calcium and its merging into bone.

Vitamin D is formed in the skin from exposure to sunlight and is available in the diet in dairy products, many of which are fortified with vitamin D, and in fish oils that are rich in vitamin D. In some areas, a lack of winter sunlight to aid in the formation of vitamin D contributes greatly to the deficiency; however, regular doses of cod liver oil, available in capsules, can overcome the problem.

rigor mortis
Stiffening of the muscles after death.

ringworm
A contagious, fungal infection of the skin.

Ringworm often appears as round patches that leave red rings; hence, its name.

Ringworm may appear in a variety of forms, on various areas of the body, as the scalp, the trunk, or the groin. Athlete's foot is also a type of ringworm.

The fungus is transmitted by direct contact with an infected person or by contact with a contaminated object, such as an article of clothing, a towel, or a hair brush. Such personal items should be discarded or cleaned with a detergent to prevent spread of the infection.

Although ringworm is more of an inconvenience than a threat, it is similar to other skin infections that may be more serious and therefore should be referred to a physician.

Rocky Mountain spotted fever
An infectious disease transmitted by wood ticks.

The microorganism that causes Rocky Mountain spotted fever is a parasite harbored by small animals, such as, dogs, rabbits, chipmunks, squirrels, etc., from which it is spread to man. Despite its name, the disease is not limited to the Rocky Mountain area, but may occur in other parts of the United States, and in other countries as well.

Infection produces chills and fever, painful muscles

and joints, and skin eruptions.

rosacea

A chronic disease characterized by reddening of the facial skin and often accompanied by pustules.

In severe cases, the nose may become red, swollen, and marked by large pores and blood vessels near the surface of the skin.

Cause of the condition is uncertain, but it has been linked to excessive consumption of caffeine in coffee, tea, cola, etc., and alcohol.

rubella

A mild, contagious, viral infection; German measles.

The onset of rubella is characterized by a runny nose, swollen glands in the neck, and a low grade fever. Small red spots become visible on the face and neck within a few days, then quickly disappear as the rash spreads over the entire body. The second rash also lasts only a few days, but swelling of the glands may persist for a bit longer.

The most serious problem associated with rubella is the likelihood of birth defect after the virus has been contracted during pregnancy.

rubeola See *measles*.

Saint Vitus Dance See *chorea*.

salmonella

A bacterium that is the cause of a type of food poisoning.

Salmonella is generally contracted by eating foods, such as meat, chicken or eggs, that have been contaminated with the bacteria.

The condition causes cramps, nausea and diarrhea. Although generally mild, lasting only a few days, salmonella can be extremely serious in the very young, the elderly, or one who is already ill. Such cases should be referred to a physician promptly.

sarcoma

Any of a number of malignant tumors that originate in connective tissue, such as bone or muscle.

scabies

A contagious skin disease caused by a burrowing mite.

Intense itching is induced by the mite burrowing into the skin to lay her eggs, generally in the area of the wrist, fingers, genitals or feet.

Medication is available to relieve itching and promote healing. The disease may be spread by close contact; therefore, anyone associating with an infested person should be treated for the condition as well.

scarlet fever

A highly contagious bacterial infection.

Scarlet fever gets its name from a characteristic scarlet rash covering the body that accompanies the fever and sore throat.

The condition is customarily treated with antibiotics accompanied by bed rest and a diet that contains lots of fluids.

scar tissue

Connective tissue that has formed to replace normal tissue damaged by disease or injury.

schizophrenia

A type of mental illness characterized by a withdrawal from reality.

Schizophrenia generally begins in adolescents or

young adults, and may be evidenced by withdrawal, hallucinations, or discussions with a nonexistent third party with references to the subject as though he or she were not there.

sciatica

Descriptive of severe pain in the lower back extending along the path followed by the sciatic nerve down the length of the back of the thigh.

scoliosis

An abnormal curvature of the spine.

Usually, the condition occurs late in life, resulting from disease of the bones or muscles supporting the spinal column; however, it may be a congenital malformation of the vertebrae that can be corrected, at least in part, by surgery.

scurvy

A disease caused by a deficiency of vitamin C.

Vitamin C performs a number of functions for the body, but is especially important in the formation of connective tissue that seals wounds, the activation of enzymes important to healing, and the prevention of clotting.

The more serious symptoms of scurvy such as anemia, general weakness, and internal hemorrhaging that can be attributed to a vitamin C deficiency are rare today, but the more obvious symptoms such as bleeding gums and slow healing are not.

Vitamin C cannot be synthesized, it is not stored in the body, and is often destroyed by other substances, such as certain medications or drugs; therefore, it should be a regular part of the diet or taken as a dietary supplement.

sebaceous cyst

A swelling formed by the retention of sebum when the duct of a sebaceous gland is obstructed.

The sebaceous glands secrete sebum, an oily substance, that aids in protecting the skin. A gland that continues to produce sebum when the duct is blocked, fills and becomes distended with the substance. Frequently, the cyst will infect, burst, and expel its contents; one that does not can be surgically removed.

seizure

A sudden attack of any kind, as by an epileptic fit, heart attack, convulsions, or a stroke.

senility

A condition that encompasses the governing factors and infirmities of old age.

Senility may be used to describe simply the condition of being old, but is more often used to express infirmities, especially the decline in mental faculties.

Senility may be characterized by memory lapse, especially for recent events; slowed speech; inability to concentrate; lethargy; lack of concern about personal appearance; lack of ability to perform routine daily tasks; loss of appetite; anxiety; insensitivity to others; irritability; or withdrawal. Severe mental decline may be manifest in impulsive or inappropriate behavior; incontinence; inability to walk; etc.

In general, these conditions are progressive, that is, once begun, they continue to worsen, a decline that may be rapid or extend over a period of many years.

septic

Descriptive of that in which bacteria or other

infectious substance is present.

shingles

A painful viral infection of the nerves; herpes zoster. Caused by the same virus as chicken pox, shingles is characterized by itching, painful blistering along the course of the infected nerve.

Treatment for shingles involves mainly medication to reduce the pain, and warm baths to bath the skin and prevent infection.

shin splints

A painful condition caused by swelling and inflamation of the membrane that joins the muscle along the lower leg bone to the bone. Shin splints are commonly a runner's affliction caused by running on a hard surface or failing to warm up properly.

shock

Shock is the failure of the *cardiovascular system,* the system that circulates blood to all cells, to provide adequate blood to every part of the body.

The collapse of the cardiovascular system may be caused by any of three conditions: blood is lost due to hemorrhaging; vessels dilate and there is insufficient blood to fill them; the heart fails to act properly as a pump and circulate the blood.

No matter what the reason for the collapse, the results are the same: an insufficient blood flow to provide adequate nourishment and oxygen to all parts of the body. The body process may slow down, reducing circulation and, without nourishment, organs begin to die, especially the brain.

The state of shock may develop rapidly or it may be delayed until hours after the event that triggers it.

shock (cont.)

Shock occurs to some degree after every injury. It may be so slight as not to be noticed; or so serious that it results in death.

Some of the major causes of shock are: severe or extensive injuries; severe pain; loss of blood; severe burns; electrical shock; certain illnesses; allergic reactions; poisoning inhaled, ingested, or injected; exposure to extremes of heat and cold; emotional stress; or substance abuse.

The signs and symptoms of shock are both physical and emotional: dazed look; paleness in light skinned individuals and ashen or grayish color in dark skinned individuals; nausea and vomiting; thirst; weak, rapid pulse; cold, clammy skin; shallow, irregular, labored breathing; pupils dilated; eyes dull and lackluster; cyanosis, or a bluish tinge to the skin, in the late stages of shock.

The most important reaction that occurs in shock is a decided drop in normal blood flow, believed to be caused by the involuntary nervous system losing control over certain small blood vessels in the abdominal cavity. This is one of the reasons the victim is nauseous.

As a large amount of blood fills the dilated vessels within the body, decreased circulation near the surface causes the skin to become pale, cold, and clammy. Other areas suffer as a result of the drop in circulation; the eyes are dull and lackluster and pupils may be dilated.

In the body's effort to fill the dilated blood vessels, less blood returns to the heart for recirculation. To overcome the decreased volume and still send blood to all parts of the body, the heart pumps faster but pumps a much lower quantity of blood per beat. Therefore, the pulse is rapid and weak.

The brain suffers from this decreased blood supply and does not function normally; the victim's powers of reasoning, thinking, and expression are dulled. The victim may exhibit: weakness and helplessness; anxiety; disorientation or confusion; or unconsciousness, in the late stages of shock.

SIDS See *crib death*.

sigmoidectomy

Surgical removal of the final section of the large intestine that connects to the rectum.

sinusitis

Inflammation of the sinus.

The sinuses are cavities in the bones of the face that are lined with mucous membrane. Normally, they are kept clear by draining into the nasal passages, but if there is any obstruction to the passage of mucus, they may become infected.

Commonly, sinusitis is associated with congestion from allergies, cold, or flu, but infection may also be caused by injury, swimming, or an abscessed tooth.

Symptoms of the infection vary, but they are often similar to the cold or flu: congestion, chills, fever, sore throat, and headache. For some sufferers, the most incapacitating symptom is a characteristic, severe headache that causes pain about the back of the head and the eyes. The sinus itself may appear puffy and swollen, and be tender to the touch.

Medication and moist heat are the most effective means for promoting drainage to relieve the pressure and remove the source of the infection. In extreme cases, surgery may be necessary to correct the condition.

skeleton

The framework of bone that supports the softer body parts.

The human skeleton is composed of approximately two hundred bones, classified according to shape as long, short, flat, and irregular. The skeleton forms a strong flexible framework for the body. It supports and carries the soft parts, protects vital organs from injury, gives attachment to muscles and tendons, and forms joints to allow movement.

There are three major divisions of the human skeleton: the *head*, *trunk*, and *extremities*.

skin

The external covering of the body.

The outer layer of skin, or epidermis, is made up of layers of cells that primarily serve to protect and also contains the cells that determine skin color. The epidermis constantly changes; as new layers are formed, old ones are shed. The layer of skin below the epidermis is the dermis. The dermis contains the blood vessels, nerves, and specialized structures such as sweat glands, that help to regulate body temperature, and hair follicles. The fat and soft tissue layer below the dermis is called the subcutaneous.

sleep

A natural state of rest characterized by a lack of voluntary thought or movement.

During sleep, the body passes through a number of

alternating states between that of being almost awake and of REM, or rapid eye movement, that is deep sleep.

It is during REM sleep, so named because of the characteristic erratic movements of the eyeballs, that dreams occur.

sleep apnea

A stoppage of breathing during sleep.

slipped disk

Descriptive of protrusion of any of the disks that cushion the vertebrae, or bones of the spinal column; a herniated disk.

The term slipped disk is a misnomer; the disk is actually herneated in that it bulges out from between the vertebrae.

smallpox

A highly contagious viral disease.

Smallpox is characterized by high fever and the emergence of red spots, first on the face and then spreading to the entire upper body. After a day or two, the spots become pustules that may leave pockmarks on the face or neck.

Although it was once a leading causes of death throughout the world, smallpox has been virtually eradicated.

smell

Descriptive of the function of the olfactory nerves; to detect odor or aroma.

sneeze

An involuntary action characterized by the sudden emission of air forcibly through the nose and mouth; a protective mechanism for expelling irritants from

spasm

the respiratory system.

spasm

The sudden, involuntary contraction of a muscle, that may be repeated for a time.

speech

The ability to create unique sounds for the sole purpose of communicating thought.

sphygmomanometer

Any device used for measuring blood pressure.

The most common sphygmomanometer is a device with an inflatable cuff that is wrapped around the subject's arm and a gauge to indicate pressure.

Blood pressure is expressed as two readings: the *systolic* that is the pressure during a contraction of the heart; and the *diastolic* that is the pressure between beats. The cuff is inflated to stop the flow of blood through the artery and then gradually deflated so that with the use of a stethoscope, the physician can determine the pressure at which the first pulse is heard and, as the cuff continues to deflate, the pressure at which the stream of blood passing through the artery is heard. Normal adult pressure is about 120/80 although some variance from that standard is not abnormal. Both readings are of value to the physician in making a diagnosis.

spinal column

The spinal column, or backbone, is made up of thirty-three segments composed of **vertebrae** joined by strong **ligaments** and **cartilage** to form a flexible column that encloses the **spinal cord**.

spinal cord

The network of nerve tissue that extends through

the spinal column.

Nerves leaving the brain connect to the spinal cord, pass down through the spinal column, the opening in the center of the spine, and branch off to all parts and organs of the body.

There are mainly two types of nerves entering and leaving the spinal cord: sensory nerves that convey sensations such as heat, cold, pain, and touch from different parts of the body to the brain; and motor nerves that convey impulses from the brain to the muscles causing movement.

spine

The human spine consists of 29 bones, called vertebrae, that provide the basis of a firm, flexible frame for the trunk of the body, and encases the spinal cord and its nerve roots.

The spinal vertebrae are separated and protected from each other by disks of cartilage that absorb the impact of any stress on the vertebrae as in walking or running.

spleen

An abdominal organ that has several functions, primarily those of removing worn out or abnormal blood cells from circulation and in the manufacture of antibodies.

spondylosis

Deterioration of the disks that separate the vertebrae of the spinal column, a condition of aging. Although most cases cause little or no discomfort, spondylosis can result in fusion and ultimately immobilization of some the bones in the spinal column.

sporadic
   Recurring at irregular intervals.
sporotrichosis
   A chronic infection caused by a fungus that exists in soil and decaying vegetation.
   Sporotrichosis commonly enters the body through ingestion or inhalation. The infection is usually limited to eruptions on the skin, but may involve the lymph glands.
sprain
   An injury due to stretching or tearing ligaments or other tissues at a joint.
   A sprain is caused by a sudden twist or stretch of a joint beyond its normal range of motion. It may be a minor injury, causing pain and discomfort for only a few hours, or it may require weeks of medical care before normal use is restored.
   A sprain is manifested by pain on movement, swelling, tenderness, and discoloration. At first the joint will probably be more comfortable if it is bandaged to limit movement and help keep the swelling down, but as soon as possible the joint should be moved and used.
   Sprains present basically the same signs as a closed fracture. If it is not possible to determine whether an injury is a fracture or a sprain, it should be treated as a fracture and referred to a physician.
spur
   A pointed outgrowth on a bone, caused by illness or injury.
sputum
   Saliva, often mixed with other material, as mucus,

that is spit from the mouth.

Excess mucus in the respiratory tract, usually the result of irritation or infection, stimulates nerve endings that set up a cough reflex to eject the offending material.

stammer

To involuntarily hesitate or falter when speaking.

The condition is usually readily overcome by speech therapy that focuses mainly on relaxation and proper breathing.

sterilization

Any condition that inhibits or destroys reproductive capability.

Sterilization may be caused by disease, disability or surgical procedure.

In men, surgical sterilization is called a vasectomy, a relatively simple procedure that involves cutting through the tubes that carry sperm from the testes to the urethra.

In women, the most common procedure is cutting or blocking the fallopian tubes that carry the egg from the ovaries to the uterus.

sternum See *breastbone*.

stimulant

Anything that has the effect of increasing the activity of a process or organ.

stomach

The organ in the digestive system that is located between the esophagus, that delivers ingested food, and the duodenum, the first part of the small intestine. The stomach mainly churns ingested food and mixes it with digestive juices before passing it on to the duodenum for further digestion and absorption.

stomatitis

See *canker sores*.

strain

An injury to a muscle or a tendon caused by stretching or overexertion.

In severe cases muscles or tendons are torn and the muscle fibers are stretched. Strains are commonly caused by a sudden, unusual or unaccustomed movement.

A strain may cause intense pain, moderate swelling, painful or difficult movement, and, sometimes, discoloration. Generally, rest is all that is required to allow the body to replace damaged tissue; however, severe or persisting discomfort should be referred to a physician for diagnosis.

strangulation

Constriction that cuts off a vital flow, as of air to the lungs or blood to an organ.

strep throat

A bacterial infection of the throat.

Strep throat may cause chills and fever, and swelling of the lymph glands.

stress

Any force or influence that tends to distort the normal physical or mental state.

Physically, stress is produced by normal body action, as that of the vertebrae against the disks that separate them when one is walking or running, or by abnormal stimulation, such as disease, injury, extreme ambient temperatures, etc. Mentally or emotionally, a certain amount of stress is inherent in every conscious thought or decision. Stress is recognized as a condition, however, only when it is sufficiently intense as to be beyond the ability of the body's regulating mechanisms to cope with it.

Stress may be brought on by any number of conditions that vary with the individual. For most, major lifetime events, such as loss of a job or the death of a loved one may trigger an extreme response that manifests itself in the onset or worsening of a mental or physical disorder. Others may attach special importance to less significant events and overreact to them, as an adolescent who regularly suffers asthma attacks before examinations in school.

stricture

An abnormal constricting of a passage that prevents normal function.

stroke

The sudden disruption of blood supply to an area of the brain; apoplexy.

Stoke may be caused by a clot formed somewhere else in the body that travels through the bloodstream to block an artery leading to the brain or in the brain, by cerebral hemorrhage brought on by the bursting of an artery in the brain, or by rupture of an *aneurysm* in an artery leading to the brain.

Those who suffer from both *hypertension* and *atherosclerosis* are the most likely candidates for a stroke, as both conditions weaken and damage the arteries. Lifestyle can also affect one's likelihood of suffering a stroke—smoking and high cholesterol levels are both significant contributing factors.

The consequence of a stroke is the loss of function in

those areas of the body controlled by the affected area of the brain. Such loss of function, such as memory, sensory perception or motor skills, may be temporary, or it may be permanent.

sty

A common infection of the sebaceous gland of the eyelash.

The sebaceous glands secrete sebum, an oily substance that aids in protecting the skin. The gland may become infected and pass the infection on to the hair follicle to which it is attached. The infection causes redness, swelling, and often, tenderness in the area. The sty may mature and burst, expelling its contents.

A sty will normally run its course without special treatment. Discomfort may be eased by relaxing the eye with occasional warm compresses and by wearing dark glasses. A child with a sty should be cautioned against touching or rubbing the eye and warned of the possibility that matter from the eye may dry during sleep, making the eyelid difficult to open on awakening—a frightening experience. In such cases, the matter is easily dissolved with a warm, moist compress.

subconscious

Descriptive of those mental processes that occur without conscious recognition or with reduced perception, as those that are instinctive or reactive.

subdural hematoma

A blood clot in the skull, beneath the outer covering of the brain

sublimation
   The suppression of base instincts to adapt to socially acceptable behavior.
subliminal
   Descriptive of that which is below the level of consciousness.
sudden death
   The immediate and unexpected cessation of respiration and functional circulation.

   The term *sudden death* is synonymous with cardiopulmonary arrest or heart-lung arrest. In the definition, the terms *sudden and unexpected* are extremely important. The death of a person with an organic disease such as cancer, or who is under treatment for a chronic heart condition and has gradual but progressive loss of heart function, cannot be correctly classified as *sudden death*. Cardiac arrest, when the heart stops pumping blood, may occur suddenly and unexpectedly for any number of reasons, such as heart attack, electric shock, asphyxiation, suffocation, drowning, allergic reaction, choking, or severe injury

   A person is considered clinically dead the moment the heart stops beating and breathing ceases. However, the vital centers of the central nervous system within the brain may remain viable for four to six minutes more. Irreversible brain damage begins to occur to human brain cells somewhere between four and six minutes after oxygen has been excluded. This condition is referred to as biological death. Resuscitation in the treatment of sudden death depends upon this grace period of four to six minutes.

After that period, even though the heart might yet be restarted, the chance of return to a normal functional existence is lessened.

sudden infant death syndrome See *crib death*.

suffocation
Any condition that inhibits the flow of air into the lungs.

suicide
The conscious taking of one's own life.

sunburn
Inflammation and discoloration of the skin caused by excessive exposure to ultraviolet rays of the sun. . Despite the extreme discomfort of sunburn, most cases need only be treated with applications of medicated ointment to help restore the moisture balance in the skin. Extreme cases, however, can involve serious damage to the skin and loss of body moisture. Any sunburn victim who suffers from chills, fever, or nausea should be placed in the care of a physician. Regular exposure to the ultraviolet rays of the sun has been linked to cancer and other skin diseases; therefore, one who is subject to such exposure should consider the use of a sun blocking lotion for protection.

superficial
Near the surface; descriptive of that which expresses only limited intrusion, as a superficial wound.

suppurative
Descriptive of the formation or presence of pus, as in a wound.

suture
To join together the edges of an open wound by

stitching; the stitch used to join the edges of a wound.

symptom
A characteristic indicator of a disease or infection, either evident to the examiner or a sensation described by the subject, that, taken with other indicators, forms the basis for a diagnosis.

syncope
Loss of consciousness caused by a temporary interruption in the flow of blood to the brain; fainting.

syndrome
A number of indicators that, taken together, form a pattern for diagnosis.

synesthesia
The alteration or transference of impressions from one sense to another, commonly that of smell or taste perceived as a visual color image.

synovial fluid
The fluid present in the joints to lubricate the synovial membrane.

synovial membrane
The membrane of the joints that, with synovial fluid, reduces the friction between two or more joined bones.

tachycardia
Abnormally rapid heartbeat, caused by disease, medication, drugs, exercise, or emotional distress.

tantrum
Uncontrollable rage or temper.

tapeworm
A long, thin, flat worm that survives in the intestinal tract.

taste

Tapeworms can cause weight loss and anemia in spite of a healthy appetite

taste

That one of the senses stimulated by contact with the tastes buds in the mouth.

Basically, the taste buds allow one to distinguish among four different characteristics—sweet, sour or acid, salty and bitter. The distinctive taste of a specific substance is a combination of the sensory perception of the taste buds, its aroma, and its texture.

tendinitis

Inflammation of a tendon.

Although tendinitis may be associated with disease, it is most usually the result of physical activity.

One who engages in athletics or physical labor without proper conditioning or preparation is a candidate for a variety of injuries, including tendinitis.

Tendinitis is manifested in pain and tenderness in the affected area, which is relieved by resting.

tendon

The tough, fibrous connective tissue by which muscle is joined to bone.

teratoma

A tumor comprised of embryonic tissue.

tetanus

An infectious disease associated with severe muscle contraction; lockjaw

The tetanus bacteria enter the body through an open wound and produce a toxin that commonly infects the muscles of the jaw, producing steady contractions that cause the jaw to become fixed in a tightly closed position.

The disease may affect other muscles, as well, and in some cases, the contractions become so severe that they are extremely painful.

The disease may be treated with drugs to counteract the infection and others to relax the muscles.

Prevention requires prompt cleansing of puncture wounds and immunization with the tetanus vaccine.

tetany

A disease caused by a lack of calcium in the blood.

Tetany is commonly associated with parathyroid disease or a lack of vitamin D in the diet. The condition causes muscle spasms and violent twitching, especially of the extremities.

thalamus

A part of the brain involved in the transmission of sensory messages.

therapeutics

The branch of medicine concerned with the treatment of disease.

thermography

A technique for determining variance in temperature with the aid of an infrared camera.

Infrared rays from a source vary with the amount of heat given off. An infrared camera, capable of photographing infrared ray patterns, can produce an image showing the relative amounts of infrared emitted from various areas, thus allowing a diagnostician to detect areas of abnormal growth or activity.

thiamine See *vitamin B complex*.

thirst

An intuitive desire for fluid.

In order to maintain normal function, the body

thoracotomy

needs constant replenishment of fluids to replace that lost through the action of the lungs, sweat glands and kidneys. A number of conditions, such as stress, heavy exercise, or hemorrhage or disease can increase the need.

The need for fluids is signaled by a dry feeling in the throat and mouth, because moisture evaporates rapidly from those areas when the body lacks water.

thoracotomy

A surgical opening of the chest, or thorax, for diagnostic purposes or for corrective surgery.

throat

That portion of the digestive tract that forms a passage from the nose and mouth to the esophagus that leads to the stomach and the trachea that leads to the lungs.

thrombosis

Coagulation of blood; the process of forming a blood clot in the heart or a blood vessel.

thrombus

A blood clot that forms in the heart or a blood vessel.

thrush

A fungal infection, most often affecting children, that is characterized by the formation of white patches and ulcers on the mouth and throat.

thymus

A lymph gland located in the upper part of the chest cavity, or thorax; thymus gland.

thyroid gland

A gland located in front of the throat that secretes hormones for regulating the body's development and metabolism.

Thyroid hormone is involved in a number of processes throughout the body, such as the regulation of body temperature, growth, fertility, and the conversion of food to energy.

tic

An intermittent, involuntary spasm or twitch, usually of the facial muscles.

tick

Any of a number of parasitic mites that feed on the blood of their host.

Ticks attach themselves to the skin of humans and animals, carrying and transmitting a number of diseases, such as Rocky Mountain spotted fever.

To avoid further damage to body tissue and the risk of infection, a tick should not be pulled or rubbed off; removal is best accomplished by covering it with salad oil or by touching it with a lighted cigarette that will cause it to back off.

tinnea See *ringworm*.

tinnitus

A buzzing or ringing in the ear.

Tinnitus may be caused by blockage of the Eustachian tubes, excessive wax in the ears, or a disorder of the auditory nerves.

tissue

Any of a number of distinctive materials, comprised of like cells, that make up the structures of the body, such as connective tissue.

tonsillectomy

A surgical procedure for the removal of the tonsils.

tonsillitis

Infection or inflammation of the tonsils.

topical

The tonsils are two small, lymph glands located on each side of the throat at the back of the mouth. Tonsillitis is usually evidenced by a sore throat, fever and difficulty in swallowing. Often, there is evidence of swelling and inflammation of the organ. Treatment generally involves rest, relieving symptoms, and sometimes, antibiotics to clear the infection. The tonsils are seldom surgically removed except in extreme conditions.

topical
Descriptive of that designated for a particular part of the body, as the applying of a medication.

torso
The trunk of the human body.

torticollis
Wryneck; a contraction of the muscles on one side of the neck that causes the neck to twist and the head to incline to one side.

toxemia
A condition in which toxins are in the blood and thereby spread throughout the system.

toxin
Any of a variety of matter produced by micro-organisms that cause infection and disease in humans.

trachea
The tube that extends from the larynx to the bronchi in the respiratory tract; the windpipe.

tracheotomy
A surgical incision in the front of the neck into the trachea.

A tracheotomy is performed when injury or disease

causes an obstruction in the windpipe or makes it necessary to remove the larynx.

transplant

To transfer an organ or tissue; the organ or tissue so transferred.

Transplants range from those of the cornea of the eye, to skin grafts, to those of organs and tissues, many yet in the experimental stage.

The overriding problem with transplants is one of rejection—the body's immune system builds antibodies to destroy the unfamiliar tissue—so that immunosuppressive drugs are necessary to suspend this reaction. There is danger also in the use of such drugs as they make the body vulnerable to other infection that can be life threatening.

The cornea carries no blood, and so poses no threat; the grafting of skin from one part of the body to another part of the same body poses no threat. One of the more common transplants, that of a kidney, has been most successful when the donor is a close relative who most nearly matches the tissue of the recipient.

The transplant of other organs, such as the heart, liver, or pancreas, have been undertaken with mixed results. There have been transplants of artificial devices, and even organs or tissue from other species. Undoubtedly, there will be failures, but undoubtedly, too, there will be great successes.

trauma

A sudden affliction, either physical or psychological. In the practice of medicine, *trauma* is generally descriptive of physical injury or the physical symptoms

tremor

of *shock*.

In psychiatry, it is used to describe a distressing emotional experience that is difficult for the subject to deal with, and that may produce a lasting effect, as neurosis.

tremor

An involuntary shaking of a part of the body.

triage

A system of assigning a priority to the treatment of victims in a medical emergency based on such factors as urgent need and the chance for survival.

trunk

The main part of the human body comprising all except the *head* and the *extremities*. The trunk is divided into upper and lower parts by a muscular partition known as the *diaphragm*.

The upper portion of the trunk is the *chest*, its cavity, and organs. The chest is formed by twenty-four ribs, twelve on each side, that are attached in the back to vertebrae. The seven upper pairs of ribs are attached to the breastbone in front by cartilage. The next three pairs of ribs are attached in front by a common cartilage to the seventh rib instead of the breastbone. The lower two pairs of ribs, known as the floating ribs, are not attached in front.

The lower part of the trunk is the *abdomen*, its cavity, and organs. The pelvis is a basin-shaped bony structure at the lower portion of the trunk below the movable vertebrae of the spinal column, which it supports, and above the lower limbs, upon which it rests. The pelvis forms the floor of the abdominal cavity and provides deep sockets in which the heads of the thigh bones fit.

tuberculosis

A bacterial infection characterized by the formation of tubercles.

The body's immune system cannot destroy the bacterium that cause tuberculosis; therefore it encloses them in small nodules called tubercles. As a result, the invading organism remains in the body, although it is prevented from causing infection.

The majority of those infected by tuberculosis will not experience symptoms, as the bacteria remain dormant in the body. Of those who do experience symptoms, not all will do so immediately after being infected. In many cases, the tuberculosis lies dormant and becomes active only when the body is weakened by some other disease.

Tuberculosis usually acts on the lungs, but it can infect other parts of the body, such as the kidneys, spine, or digestive tract.

Tuberculosis is contagious, spread by bacteria from the coughing or sneezing of an infected person. Anyone in contact with a tuberculosis sufferer should consult a physician for testing.

The symptoms of tuberculosis are not distinctive from other infections—in the early stages, they involve fever, fatigue and weight loss; later there may be chest pains, shortness of breath and spots of blood in coughed up sputum—however, any signs of blood in the lungs should be referred to a physician regardless of the suspected cause.

tumor

Any growth of new tissue that is independent of its

surroundings. A tumor may be **benign** or **malignant**.

turgid

Descriptive of that which is swollen or abnormally distended.

ulcer

Descriptive of an erosion, or open sore; any area of skin or mucous membrane that is lacking its normal protective cover and, usually, is inflamed.

Ulcers may occur as **bedsores** on the lower back caused by extended confinement to bed, as sores of the feet or legs associated with diabetes or varicose veins, in the digestive tract such as a **peptic ulcer**, etc.

ultrasound

The technique of using high frequency sound waves to record an image of internal tissue that cannot be detected by X rays.

The sound waves are focused into beams that are deflected differently by tissues of varying density so that the existence and position of the tissue can be recorded to produce a visual image.

Ultrasound is a valuable tool in detection and diagnosis, such as the formation and position of gallstones, or irregularities in blood vessels. It can also be used for examination of the fetus during pregnancy, as it produces no harmful emission of radiation.

undulant fever See **brucellosis**.

urinary bladder

The organ or sac that receives, holds, and discharges urine.

urology

The branch of medicine that deals with the study, diagnosis and treatment of diseases and disorders of the urogenital tract, or the urinary tract and reproductive system.

urticaria

An allergic condition characterized by itchy blotches or welts; hives.

Urticaria may be caused by allergens in food, as tomatoes, strawberries, etc.; certain drugs; bacteria; animal hair; or the environment, as exposure to cold or the sun.

An outbreak may last less than an hour or continue for weeks, often subsiding, then reappearing from time to time. A mild attack is merely annoying, but more serious attacks may be accompanied by fever or nausea and even difficulty in breathing if the respiratory tract is infected. Treatment generally involves administering antihistamines.

varicose veins

A condition characterized by swollen, knotted blood vessels, usually in the legs.

Blood returning to the heart from the legs is pushed against gravity; therefore, the veins in the legs have a special valve to keep the blood from running backward. If a vein is weakened from obesity, lack of exercise, long stretches of sitting or standing, etc., it stretches and the valves are not allowed to close properly. Blood then leaks backward and gathers in pools that further weaken the vein.

Varicose veins may be temporary, as in the case of pregnancy when they are caused by the strain of carrying the additional weight, or when long periods of sitting or standing are not part of the normal lifestyle. In such cases, resumption of normal activity and exercise may help them to return to normal.

The condition is obvious, as it develops close to the skin and appears as twisting, bulging lines that run down the legs, often with dark blue spots or sections. Often the ankles swell and the skin in the affected area becomes dry and itchy. In severe cases there may be shooting pains and cramps, especially at night.

Varicose veins are not necessarily serious in themselves, but they may allow the formation of clots or inflammation that can lead to more serious problems in the future.

vasculitis
An inflammation of a blood vessel.

vein
Any of the numerous vessels that carry blood back to the heart

vertebrae
The bones or segments that make up the spinal column and through which the spinal cord passes. *Vertebrae* is plural; *vertebra* is singular.

vertigo
A disorder in which dizziness is accompanied by a sensation of moving and the feeling that one's surroundings are moving as well.

virulent
Descriptive of that which can overcome the body's defenses and cause infection; often powerful and rapid in its advance; malignant.

vitamin

Any of a number of organic substances that are essential for the normal growth and functioning of the body.

Most vitamins are derived from various food sources and some are synthesized in the body.

vitamin A

Obtained primarily from green leafy vegetables, eggs, butter, milk, liver, and fish liver oils, vitamin A is essential to proper formation of cells of the skin and mucous membranes, and for night vision.

vitamin B complex

B vitamins are divided into several constituents:

Thiamine, or *Vitamin B$_1$* is available mainly in yeast, whole grain, meat, eggs, and potato. Thiamine is important to promote growth and in the proper functioning of nerves.

Riboflavin, or *Vitamin B$_2$* may be obtained from milk, eggs, cheese, liver, and meats; it promotes growth and aids in the body cells' metabolism.

Vitamin B$_6$ is contained in whole grains, fish, liver, and yeast. It is important in the metabolism of protein and the production of antibodies to fight infection.

Vitamin B$_{12}$ is available from milk, eggs, liver and meat. It is important in the metabolism of fat and sugar; in the production of blood; and for normal growth and neurological function.

Niacin, or *nicotinic acid*, that is obtainable from yeast, liver, meat, and whole grains, aids in the metabolism of sugar and is vital to proper function of the intestines.

Vitamin C

Folic acid, obtained from green leafy vegetables, giblets, and liver, aids in the metabolism of sugar and amino acids, the components of protein.
Pantothenic acid, obtainable from green leafy vegetables and meat, is essential to cell growth.
Biotin, found in yeast, egg and liver is essential for normal growth.
Choline, found in green leafy vegetables and meat, is essential to the metabolism of fat.
Inositol, from green leafy vegetables and meat, is linked to the metabolism of cholesterol

Vitamin C

Vitamin C, or *ascorbic acid* is obtained mainly from citrus fruit, such as oranges, lemons or grapefruit, and from potatoes or tomatoes. Vitamin C is vital to the function of blood vessels, healing and the production of connective tissue.

Vitamin D

Found mainly in fish liver oil and in fortified milk, vitamin D can also be formed on the skin from sunlight. It is essential to the metabolism of calcium and important to normal formation of teeth and bones.

Vitamin E

Obtained from cold-pressed oils, wheat germ and whole grains, vitamin E is linked to a number of functions in the body including the manufacture of blood and to fertility.

Vitamin K

Available from leafy green vegetables and fish, vitamin K is necessary for the blood to clot normally.

vitiligo

A condition in which there is an absence of natural

pigment in sections of the skin or hair that appear as whitish or light patches.

vomit

To expel the contents of the stomach forcibly through the mouth.

wart

A small, dry growth on the skin.

A wart is not malignant or, in most cases, harmful in any other way. The condition is caused by a virus that causes enlargement of the cells of the skin.

wean

To teach a baby to consume foods other than mother's milk or formula.

wheeze

Difficulty in breathing that is accompanied by a whistling sound.

whooping cough

An infectious disease of the respiratory system that affects the mucous membranes lining the air passages. Primarily a disease of children, it is characterized by a series of coughs followed by an intake of breath that causes a whooping sound.

X rays

High frequency electromagnetic radiation that is capable of penetrating some solid objects, of destroying tissue by extended exposure, and of creating an image on a photographic plate or a fluorescent screen.

X rays are used to create images of body parts for study and diagnosis.

yellow fever

An often fatal viral infection contracted by the bite of an infected mosquito.

yellow jaundice.

Yellow fever attacks the liver and kidneys, and causes chills, fever, jaundice, and internal hemorrhaging.

yellow jaundice See *jaundice*.

zoonosis

Any disease in animals that can be transmitted to man.

zoster

Herpes zoster. See *shingles*.

Directory of Health Organizations

Following is a select group of organizations that may be contacted for information or assistance.

General Information

American Red Cross .... (908) 737-8300
Centers for Disease Control and Prevention
.... (404) 639-3492
Food and Drug Administration .... (301) 295-8228

Acupuncture

American Academy of Medical Acupuncture
.... (510) 841-3250

Aging

American Association of Retired Persons (AARP)
.... (202) 434-2277
American Geriatric Society .... (212) 308-1414
American Society on Aging .... (415) 882-2910
National Council of Senior Citizens, Inc.
.... (301) 578-8800
The National Council on Aging .... (202) 479-1200
National Institute on Aging .... (301) 496-1752

AIDS/HIV

AIDS Hotline .... (800) 342-AIDS
Women's AIDS Network .... (415) 621-4160
National AIDS Information Clearinghouse
.... (800) 458-5231

Alcoholism

Al-Anon Family Group .... (804) 563-1600
Alcoholics Anonymous .... (212) 870-3400

HEALTH ORGANIZATIONS

Allergies
Asthma and Allergy Foundation of America
.... (202) 466-7643
National Institute of Allergy and Infectious Disease
.... (301) 496-5717

Arthritis
The Arthritis Foundation .... (404) 237-8771
National Institute of Arthritis and Musculoskeletal
and Skin Diseases .... (301) 495-4484

Autism
Autism Society of America .... (301) 657-0881

Birth Defects
March of Dimes/Birth Defects Foundation
.... (914) 428-7100
National Institute of Child Health and Human Development .... (301) 496-5133

Blood Diseases
Leukemia Society of America, Inc (212) 573-8484
National Hemophilia Foundation... (212) 219-8180

Bone and Muscular Disorders
National Institute of Arthritis and Musculoskeletal
and Skin Diseases .... (301) 495-4484
National Osteoporosis Foundation (202) 223-2226

Cancer
American Cancer Society, Inc. .... (404) 320-3333
Cancer Counseling and Research Center
.... (500) 686-6000
Cancer Information Clearinghouse (800) 4-CANCER
Ronald McDonald Houses .... (312) 836-7100

Cardiovascular Disease

American Heart Association .... (214) 373-6300
National Heart, Lung, and Blood Institute
.... (301) 496-4236
The Sister Kenny Institute .... (612) 863-4457

Cerebral Palsy

United Cerebral Palsy Association, Inc.
.... (212) 979-9700
National Institute of Neurological Disorders and
Stroke .... (800) 352-9424

Child Abuse and Neglect

National Clearinghouse for Child Abuse and Neglect
Information .... (800) FYI-3366
National Child Abuse Hotline ...... (800) 422-4453
National Council on Child Abuse and Family
Violence .... (202) 429-6695

Chiropractic

American Chiropractic Association (703) 276-8800

Cystic Fibrosis

Cystic Fibrosis Foundation .... (800) 344-4823

Diabetes

American Diabetes Association ... (212) 725-4925
National Diabetes Information Clearinghouse (301)
654-3327

Down Syndrome and Mental Retardation

National Down Syndrome Society (800) 221-4602
American Association on Mental Retardation
.... (202) 387-1968
Association for Retarded Citizens (817) 261-6003
Kennedy Child Study Center .... (212) 988-9500

Drug and Alcohol Abuse

Mothers Against Drunk Driving (MADD)
.... (800) 438-MADD
National Association for Children of Alcoholics, Inc.
.... (301) 468-0985
National Clearinghouse for Alcohol and Drug Information .... (301) 468-2600
National Council on Alcoholism and Drug Dependence, Inc. .... (800) 622-2255
National Drug Abuse and Treatment Hotline
.... (800) 662-HELP

Eating Disorders

National Institute of Mental Health (301) 443-4515

Epilepsy

Epilepsy Foundation of America .. (301) 459-3700
Epilepsy Institute .... (212) 677-8550

Family Planning/Sex Information

Planned Parenthood Federation of America, Inc.
.... (212) 541-7800
Population Council, Inc. .... (212) 339-0500

Fitness

President's Council on Physical Fitness and Sports
.... (202) 272-3430

Hearing and Speech Disorders

Alexander Graham Bell Association for the Deaf
.... (202) 337-5220
American Tinnitus Association .... (503) 248-9985
National Association of the Deaf .. (301) 587-1788
National Information Center on Deafness
.... (202) 651-5051

HEALTH ORGANIZATIONS

Herbal Medicine
The American Botanical Council . (512) 331-8868
The Herb Research Foundation ... (303) 449-2265

Home Care and Hospice
The National Association for Home Care
.... (202) 547-7424
Hospice Education Institute .... (800) 331-1620
National Hospice Organization .... (800) 658-8898

Hypnotherapy
American Council of Clinical Hypnosis
.... (312) 297-3317

Kidney Disease
National Kidney Foundation, Inc.   (800) 622-9010

Learning Disabilities
Association for Children with Learning Disabilities
.... (412) 341-1515

Massage
American Massage Therapy Association
.... (312) 761-2682

Medic Alert
Medic Alert Foundation International
.... (800) ID-ALERT

Mental Health
National Mental Health Association (703) 684-7722
National Institute of Mental Health (301) 443-4513

Neurologic Disorders
Association for Alzheimer's and Related Diseases
.... (800) 621-0379

HEALTH ORGANIZATIONS

Neuromuscular Disorders
National Multiple Sclerosis Society (212) 986-3240
Muscular Dystrophy Association of America, Inc.
.... (212) 557-8450
Myasthenia Gravis Foundation, Inc. (212) 533-7005

Nursing Homes
American Assocation of Homes for the Aging
.... (202) 783-2242
American Health Care Association (202) 842-4444

Organ Donation
The Living Bank .... (800) 528-2971
United Network for Organ Sharing (800) 24-DONOR

Pain Relief
American Chronic Pain Association, Inc.
.... (916) 632-0922

Parkinson's Disease
National Parkinson's Foundation   (800) 327-4545
.... (800) 433-7022 (in Florida)
Parkinson's Disease Foundation . (212) 923-4700
The Parkinson Support Group of America
.... (301) 937-1545
United Parkinson Foundation ..... (312) 733-1893

Rehabilitation
Disabled American Veterans .... (606) 441-7300
Federation of the Handicapped ... (212) 727-4200
Goodwill Industries of America ... (202) 636-4225
Human Resources Center .... (516) 747-5400
The National Easter Seal Society . (312) 726-6200
National Rehabilitation Association (703) 836-0850
National Rehabilitation Information Center
.... (800) 346-2742

Respiratory Disorders
American Lung Association .... (212) 889-3370
Asthma and Allergy Foundation of America
.... (202) 466-7643

Sexually Transmitted Diseases
National Sexually Transmitted Disease Hotline
.... (800) 227-8922

Smoking
Action on Smoking and Health .... (202) 659-4310
Centers for Disease Control .... (770) 488-5705
Smokenders .... (800) 828-4357

Sudden Infant Death Syndrome (SIDS)
Sudden Infant Death Syndrome (SIDS) Resource
Center .... (703) 821-8955 Ext. 249

Surgery
American College of Surgeons ..... (312) 644-4030
American Society of Plastic and Reconstructive
Surgeons .... (708) 228-9900
Non-Emergency Surgery Hotline . (800) 638-6833

Travelers
Centers for Disease Control and Prevention
.... (404) 332-4555
Health Guide for Travelers .... (800) 237-6615
Runaway Hotline .... (800) 231-6946

Urinary Tract Disorders
American Foundation for Urologic Disease
.... (800) 242-AFUD
Continence Restored, Inc. .... (212) 879-3131
Help for Incontinent People .... (800) BLADDER

Visual Impairment

American Council for the Blind ... (800) 424-8666
American Printing House for the Blind
.... (502) 895-2405
Fight for Sight .... (212) 751-1118
Guiding Eyes for the Blind, Inc. .. (914) 245-4024
National Eye Institute .... (301) 496-5248
Recording for the Blind, Inc. .... (609) 452-0606
The Seeing Eye, Inc. .... (201) 539-4425

Women's Health

National Women's Health Network (202) 347-1140

Emergency First Aid Guide

Contents

Importance of First Aid

Sudden illness or injury can often be serious unless proper care is administered promptly. **First aid** is immediate attention to one suffering from illness or injury.

First aid does not replace the physician, but assists the victim until proper medical assistance can be obtained. One of the most important principles of first aid is to obtain medical assistance in all cases of serious injury. Even seemingly minor injuries should be examined by a physician if there is any possibility of complication.

When first aid is properly administered, it can often restore natural breathing and circulation, control bleeding, reduce the severity of shock, protect injuries from infection or other complications, and help conserve the victim's strength. If prompt steps are taken and medical aid is obtained, the victim's chances of recovery are greatly improved.

First aiders must be able to take charge of a situation, keep calm while working under pressure, and organize others to do likewise. By demonstrating competence and using well-selected words of encouragement, first aiders should win the confidence of others nearby and do everything possible to reassure the apprehensive victim.

During the first few minutes following an injury, the injured person has a better chance of full recovery if there is someone nearby trained in first aid. Everyone should be able to give effective assistance until an injured person can receive professional medical care.

General Procedures

No two situations requiring first aid are the same; however, the following procedures are generally applicable:

- Take charge or follow instructions! If you are first at the scene, instruct someone to obtain medical help and others to assist as directed. If you arrive after someone else has taken charge, do as you are asked by the person in charge.
- Secure the scene. Ask someone to remove or mark any hazards.

FIRST AID GUIDE

- If several people have been injured, decide upon priorities in caring for each of the victims.
- Make a primary survey of the victim.
- Care for life-threatening conditions.
- Make a secondary survey of victim.
- Care for all injuries in order of need.
- Keep the injured person or persons lying down.
- Loosen restrictive clothing if necessary.
- Cover victim to keep warm and dry.
- Keep onlookers away from the victim.
- When necessary, improvise first aid materials using whatever is available.
- Cover all wounds completely.
- Prevent air from reaching burned surfaces as quickly as possible by using a suitable dressing.
- Remove small, loose foreign objects from a wound by brushing away from the wound with a piece of sterile gauze.
- **Do not** try to remove embedded objects.
- Place a bandage compress and a cover bandage over an open fracture without undue pressure before applying splints.
- Support and immobilize fractures and dislocations.
- Except for lower jaw dislocations, leave the reduction of fractures or dislocations to a doctor.
- Unless absolutely necessary, never move a victim until fractures have been immobilized.
- Test a stretcher before use, carefully place an injured person on the stretcher, and carry the victim without any unnecessary movements.

Evaluating the Situation

First aiders should take charge with full recognition of their own limitations and, while caring for life-threatening conditions, direct others briefly and clearly as to exactly what they should do and how to secure assistance. Information should be gathered to determine the extent of the injuries.

Patient Assessment

Primary Survey

Many conditions may be life-threatening, but three in particular require immediate action:

- Respiratory arrest
- Circulatory failure
- Severe bleeding

Respiratory arrest and/or circulatory failure can set off a chain of events that will lead to death.

Severe and uncontrolled bleeding can lead to an irreversible state of shock in which death is inevitable. Before caring for lesser injuries, the first aider should follow the ABC method to check for life-threatening conditions:

A) Airways—Establish responsiveness, position the victim, and ensure adequate breathing. If there are no signs of breathing, artificial ventilation must be given immediately.

B) Bleeding—Make a careful and thorough check for any bleeding. Control serious bleeding.

C) Circulation—In cases of circulatory failure, a person *trained* in cardiopulmonary resuscitation (CPR) should check for a pulse, and if none is detected, start CPR at once.

In making the primary survey, **do not** move the victim any more than is necessary. Rough handling or unnecessary movement might cause additional pain and aggravate serious injuries.

Secondary Survey

When the life-threatening conditions have been controlled, the secondary survey should begin. The secondary survey is a head-to-toe examination to check **carefully** for any additional unseen injuries that can cause serious complications. This is conducted by examining for the following:

- Neck - Examine for neck injury—tenderness, deformity, medical identification necklace, etc. Spine fractures, especially in the neck area may accompany head injuries. Gently feel and look for any abnormalities. If a spinal injury is suspected, stop the secondary survey until the head can be stabilized.
- Head - Without moving the head, check for blood in the hair, scalp lacerations, and contusions. Gently feel for possible bone fragments or depressions in the skull. Loss of fluid or bleeding from the ears and nose is an indication of possible skull fracture.
- Chest - Check the chest for cuts, impaled objects, fractures, and penetrating (sucking) wounds by observing chest movement. When the sides are not rising together or one side is not moving at all, there may be lung and rib damage.
- Abdomen - Gently feel the abdominal area for cuts, penetrations, and impaled objects; look for

spasms and tenderness.
- Lower back - Feel for deformity and tenderness.
- Pelvis - Check for grating, tenderness, bony protrusions, and depressions in the pelvic area.
- Genital region - Check for any obvious injury.
- Upper and lower extremities - Check for discoloration, swelling, tenderness, and deformities which are sometimes present with fractures and dislocations. Paralysis in the arms and legs indicates a fractured neck. Paralysis in the legs indicates a fractured back. Check for a medical identification bracelet.
- Back surfaces - Injuries underneath the victim are often overlooked. Examine for bony protrusions, bleeding, and obvious injuries.

If the victim is conscious, explain that you are going to perform the head-to-toe survey and inform him or her what you are going to do. Be reassuring at all times.

Besides being trained in proper first aid methods, all first aiders should know what first aid equipment is available at home, at work, in the car, etc. The equipment should be checked periodically.

Artificial Ventilation

Causes of Respiratory Arrest

Breathing may stop as a result of a variety of serious accidents. The most common causes are overdoses of narcotics, electric shock, drowning, suffocation, poisonous gases, head injuries, and heart problems.

Electric shock

The symptoms of electric shock are sudden loss of consciousness, impairment or absence of respiration or circulation, weak pulse, and sometimes burns. Breathing may be so weak and shallow that it cannot be detected.

If the victim is free from contact with the electric current, begin first aid at once. If the victim is still in contact with the current, rescue the victim at once, being careful not to come in contact with the current. **Every second of delay in removing a person from contact with an electric current lessens the chance of resuscitation.** In all cases, remove the current from the victim or the victim from the current promptly. Start artificial ventilation or CPR at once, if necessary.

Drowning

Remove a victim of drowning from the water as quickly as possible. Begin artificial ventilation immediately without taking the time to remove water which may be in the respiratory tract.

Drowning is a form of suffocation. The supply of air to the lungs has been cut off completely by water or spasm of the larynx. This cutoff does not create an immediate lack of oxygen in the body. There is a small reserve in the air cells of the lungs, in the blood and in some of the tissue that can sustain life for up to six minutes or longer at low temperatures. Because this reserve is exhausted relatively quickly, it is important to start artificial ventilation as soon as possible.

Suffocation

Always rescue a suffocation victim as quickly as possible. Symptoms of suffocation in an unconscious person are: the lips, fingernails, and ear lobes become blue or darker in color; the pulse becomes rapid and weak; breathing stops; and the pupils of the eyes become dilated. The cause may be a blocked windpipe preventing air from getting into the lungs. **Artificial ventilation is of no value until blockage is removed.**

Dangerous Gases

Several noxious or toxic gases encountered in everyday life can cause asphyxiation, including carbon monoxide, sulfur dioxide, oxides of nitrogen, ammonia, hydrogen cyanide, and cyanogen compounds. Persons should be aware of the early warning signs of exposure so gases may be detected before asphyxiation occurs. Headache, nausea, and tearing of the eyes are the three most common symptoms of the presence of dangerous gases. Rescuers should take care to protect themselves. Unless the surrounding air is good, take the victim to pure air immediately and begin artificial ventilation at once.
Nontoxic gases such as carbon dioxide and methane may also cause suffocation by displacing oxygen.

Principles of Artificial Ventilation

Artificial ventilation is the process for causing air flow in and out of the lungs when natural breathing has ceased or when it is irregular or inadequate.
At the top of the windpipe is a flap, the epiglottis, which closes over the windpipe during swallowing to

keep food or liquid from entering it. When a person is unconscious, the flap may fail to respond; therefore, no solids or liquids should be given by mouth, since they may enter the windpipe and lungs and cause suffocation or serious complications. If an unconscious person is lying on his or her back, the tongue is apt to fall against the back of the throat and interfere with air reaching the lungs. Sometimes it may block the throat entirely.

When a person is unconscious or breathing with difficulty, the head-tilt/chin-lift maneuver should be used to open the airway. **This procedure is not recommended for a victim with possible neck or spinal injuries.**

When breathing has ceased, the body's oxygen supply is cut off; brain cells start to die within four to six minutes. This can cause irreversible brain damage and if breathing is not restored, death will occur. In some cases the heart may continue to beat and circulate blood for a short period after a person stops breathing. If artificial ventilation is started within a short time after respiratory arrest, the victim has a good chance for survival.

Certain general principles must always be kept in mind when administering artificial ventilation by any method:

- Every second counts.
- **Do not** take time to move the victim unless the accident site is hazardous.
- **Do not** delay ventilation to loosen the victim's clothing or warm the victim. These are of secondary importance to getting air into the victim's lungs.

- Perform head-tilt/chin-lift method for opening airway, which will bring the tongue forward.
- Remove any visible foreign objects from the mouth.
- An assistant should loosen any tight fitting clothing in order to promote circulation and go or send for help.
- Use a blanket, clothing or other material to keep the victim warm and dry.
- Maintain a steady, constant rhythm while giving artificial ventilation. Be sure to look for rise and fall of the chest and look, listen, and feel for return air. If none, look for upper airway obstruction.
- Continue artificial ventilation until one of the following occurs:
    - Spontaneous breathing resumes
    - You are relieved by a qualified person
    - A doctor pronounces the victim dead
- You are exhausted and physically unable to continue
- **Do not** fight the victim's attempts to breathe.
- Once the victim recovers, constantly monitor the victim's condition because breathing may stop again.
- Keep the victim lying down.
- Treat the victim for physical shock.

Methods of Artificial Ventilation

The first thing to do when finding an unconscious person is to establish unresponsiveness by tapping on the shoulder and asking "Are you OK?" Place the victim on his or her back. Open the airway by using the head-tilt/chin-lift method. Remove any visible foreign objects from the mouth. To assess the presence or absence of spontaneous breathing in a victim, the rescuer should place his or her ear near the victim's mouth and nose while maintaining the open airway position. Look toward the victim's body and while observing the victim's chest, the rescuer should:

LOOK for the chest to rise and fall;

LISTEN for air escaping during exhalation;

FEEL for the flow of air.

If the chest does not rise and fall and no air is heard or felt, the victim is not breathing. This assessment should take only three to five seconds. If it is determined that the victim is not breathing, begin artificial ventilation.

Mouth-to-Mouth Ventilation

Mouth-to-mouth ventilation is by far the most effective means of artificial ventilation for use on a victim of respiratory arrest.

- Open the airway. The most common cause of airway obstruction in an unconscious victim is the tongue. The tongue is attached to the lower jaw; moving the jaw forward lifts the tongue away from the back of the throat and opens the airway.
  - Kneel at the victim's side with knee nearest the head opposite the victim's shoulders.
  - Use the **head-tilt/chin-lift maneuver** (if no spinal injury exists) to open airway. Place one of your hands on the fore-

head and apply gentle, firm, backward pressure using the palm of your hand. Place the fingertips of your other hand under the chin. The fingertips are used to bring the chin forward and to support the jaw.

- Pinch the nose closed. Inhale deeply and place your mouth over the victim's mouth (over mouth and nose with children) making sure of a tight seal. Give two full breaths into the air passage watching for the chest to rise after each breath.
- Keep the victim's head extended at all times.
- Remove your mouth between breaths and let the victim exhale.
- Feel and listen for the return flow of air, and look for fall of the victim's chest.

If neck injury is suspected, use modified jaw-thrust.

- Place victim on his or her back.
- Kneel at the top of victim's head, resting on your elbows.
- Reach forward and gently place one hand on each side of victim's chin, at the angles of the lower jaw.
- Push the victim's jaw forward, applying most of the pressure with your index fingers.
- **Do not** tilt or rotate the victim's head.

Repeat this procedure giving one breath twelve times per minute for an adult, fifteen times per minute for a small child. For an infant, give gentle puffs of air from the mouth twenty times per minute.

Mouth-to-Nose Ventilation

In certain cases, mouth-to-nose ventilation may be required. The mouth-to-nose technique is similar to mouth-to-mouth except that the lips are sealed by pushing the lower jaw against the upper jaw and air is forced into the victim by way of the nose.

Gastric Distention

One problem that may occur during artificial ventilation is the accumulation of air in the victim's stomach. Air in the stomach can cause two problems:

- Reduction in the volume of air that enters the lungs because the diaphragm is farther forward than normal
- Vomiting

To reduce distention, proceed as follows:

- Reposition the victim's head to provide a better airway.
- Limit ventilation force and volume.
- If vomiting occurs, turn the victim on his or her side if no spinal injury is present.
- **Do not** press on the stomach unless suction equipment is available and you have been trained to use it, otherwise material from the stomach may become lodged in the lungs.

Obstructed Airway

An obstruction in the airway can cause unconsciousness and respiratory arrest. There are many factors that can partially or fully obstruct the airway, such as gum, tobacco, or loose dentures. A variety of foods can cause choking, but meat is the most common.

When the airway is completely obstructed, the victim is unable to speak, breath, or cough and will clutch the neck. Some people will use the universal distress signal for choking—a hand raised to the neck with fingers extended around the neck in one direction, the thumb in the other direction as though attempting to choke oneself.

Conscious Victim, Sitting or Standing

- Determine if obstruction of airway is partial or complete.
- If partial obstruction, that is, there is some exchange of air, encourage victim to cough.
- If there is no air exchange, stand behind and place your arms around the victim's waist.
- Grasp one fist in your other hand and position the thumb side of your fist against the middle of the victim's abdomen just above the navel and well below the rib cage.
- **Do not** squeeze victim.
- Press your fist into the victim's abdominal area with a quick upward thrust.
- Repeat the procedure if necessary.

Chest Thrust, Conscious Victim

The chest thrust is another method of applying the manual thrust when removing an obstruction from the airway. Use this method on a pregnant victim or when the rescuer is unable to wrap his or her arms around the victim's waist, as in gross obesity.

- When the conscious victim is standing or sitting, position yourself behind him or her and slide your arms under the armpits, so that you encircle the chest.
- Make a fist with one hand and place the thumb

side of this fist on the victim's sternum.

- Make contact with the midline of the sternum about two to three finger-widths above the lower tip of the sternum.
- Grasp the fist with your other hand and press with a quick backward thrust.
- Repeat thrusts until the obstruction is expelled or the victim becomes conscious.

Victim Alone

The victim of an obstructed airway who is alone may use his or her own fist as described previously, or bend over the back of a chair and exert downward pressure.

Unconscious Victim

When you attempt to give artificial ventilation and you feel resistance, that is, the air is not getting in, the victim's airway is probably obstructed. The most common cause of airway obstruction in an unconscious person is the tongue falling back into the airway, which can be corrected by using the head-tilt/chin-lift maneuver. When the airway is obstructed by a foreign body, the obstruction must be cleared or ventilation will be ineffective.

Abdominal Thrust, Victim Lying Down

- Position victim on his or her back, face up.
- Straddle victim's hips, if possible.
- Place the heel of one hand against the middle of the victim's abdomen between the rib cage and the navel with fingers pointing toward the victim's chest.
- Place your other hand on top of the first.
- Move your shoulders directly over the victim's

abdomen.
- Press into the victim's abdominal area with a quick upward thrust.
- Do six to ten thrusts.
- Follow with opening mouth and finger sweep.
- Attempt artificial ventilation.
- Repeat the procedures until obstruction is cleared.

Chest Thrust, Victim Lying Down

Apply the chest thrust method to remove an obstruction from a pregnant or obese victim.

- Position the victim on his or her back.
- Open the airway.
- Kneel close to the victim.
- Place the heel of one hand on the lower half of the breast bone about one to one and one-half inches above the tip (xiphoid process) with fingers elevated. The heel of the hand must be parallel to the breast bone.
- Place the other hand on top of and parallel to the first hand.
- With your shoulders directly over your hands, exert a downward thrust. Keep elbows straight by locking them.
- Do six to ten thrusts.
- Follow with opening mouth and finger sweep.
- Attempt artificial ventilation.
- Repeat the procedure until obstruction is cleared.

Manual Removal

Whenever a foreign object is in the victim's mouth, the rescuer should remove it with the fingers.

Manual thrusts may dislodge the obstruction, but not expel it. The rescuer should turn the victim face up, open the victim's mouth with the cross-finger technique or tongue-jaw lift if necessary, and clear the obstruction with a finger sweep.

Tongue-Jaw Lift

Open victim's mouth by grasping both the tongue and lower jaw and lifting.

Cross-Finger Technique

- Cross your thumb under your index finger.
- Brace your thumb and finger against the victim's upper and lower teeth.
- Push your fingers apart to separate the jaws.

Finger Sweep

- Open the victim's jaws with one hand.
- Insert the index finger of your other hand down the inside of the cheek and into the throat to the base of the tongue.
- The index finger is then swept across the back of the throat in a hooking action to dislodge the obstruction.
- Grasp and remove the foreign object when it comes within reach.

Cardiopulmonary Resuscitation (CPR)

Cardiopulmonary resuscitation (CPR) involves the use of artificial ventilation (mouth-to-mouth breathing) and external heart compression (rhythmic pressure on the breastbone). **These techniques must be learned through training and supervised practice. Courses are available through the**

American Heart Association and American Red Cross. Incorrect application of external heart compressions may result in complications such as damage to internal organs, fracture of ribs or sternum, or separation of cartilage from ribs. (Rib fractures may occur when compressions are being correctly performed but this is not an indication to stop compression.) **Application of cardiopulmonary resuscitation when not required could result in cardiac arrest, so never practice these skills on another person.** When CPR is properly applied, the likelihood of complications is minimal and acceptable in comparison with the alternative—death.

Sudden Death

Sudden death is the immediate and unexpected cessation of respiration and functional circulation. The term *sudden death* is synonymous with cardiopulmonary arrest or heart-lung arrest. Cardiac arrest, when the heart stops pumping, may occur suddenly and unexpectedly for any number of reasons:

- Heart attack
- Electric shock
- Asphyxiation
- Suffocation
- Drowning
- Allergic reaction
- Choking
- Severe injury

A person is considered clinically dead the moment the heart stops beating and breathing ceases. However, the vital centers of the central nervous system within the brain may remain viable for four to six minutes more. Irreversible brain damage begins to occur to human brain cells somewhere between four and six minutes after oxygen has been excluded. This condition is referred to as biological death. Resuscitation in the treatment of sudden death depends upon this grace period of four to six minutes.

Heart Attack

Recognition of the early warning signs of an impending heart attack is extremely important:

- Uncomfortable pressure, squeezing, fullness, or dull pain in the center of the chest lasting for more than minutes
- Pain may radiate into the shoulders, arm, neck or jaw.,
- Sweating
- Nausea
- Shortness of breath
- Feeling of weakness
- Pale and sick looking

A person need not exhibit all these symptoms to have a heart attack. The symptoms of heart attack may come and go, often leading the victim to attribute them to another cause such as indigestion.

Recognizing the Problem

The person who initiates emergency heart-lung resuscitation has two responsibilities:

- To apply emergency measures to keep the clinically dead victim biologically alive
- To be sure the victim receives proper medical care

In addition to performing CPR, the rescuer must

summon help in order that an ambulance and/or a physician may be called to the scene.

CPR Procedure for Single Rescuer

The CPR procedures should be learned and practiced on a training mannequin under the guidance of a qualified instructor. The step by step procedure for cardiopulmonary resuscitation is as follows:

- **Establish unresponsiveness.** Gently shake the victim's shoulder and shout, "Are you OK?" The individual's response or lack of response will indicate to the rescuer if the victim is just sleeping or unconscious.
- **Call for help.** Help will be needed to assist in performing CPR or to call for medical help.
- **Position the victim.** If the victim is found in a crumpled up position and/or face down, the rescuer must roll the victim over; this is done while calling for help.

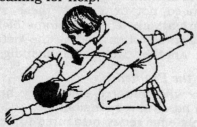

- When rolling the victim over, take care that broken bones are not further complicated by improper handling. Roll the victim as a unit so that the head, shoulders, and torso move

simultaneously with no twisting.
- Kneel beside the victim, a few inches to the side.
- The arm nearest the rescuer should be raised above the victim's head.
- The rescuer's hand closest to the victim's head should be placed on the victim's head and neck to prevent them from twisting.
- The rescuer should use the other hand to grasp under the victim's arm furthest from rescuer. This will be the point at which the rescuer exerts the pull in rolling the body over.
- Pull carefully under the arm, and the hips and torso will follow the shoulders with minimal twisting.
- Be sure to watch the neck and keep it in line with the rest of the body.
- The victim should now be flat on his or her back.
- **A-Airway. Open the airway.** The most common cause of airway obstruction in an unconscious victim is the tongue.
  - Use the head-tilt/chin-lift maneuver to open airway. (This maneuver is not recommended for a victim with possible neck or spinal injuries.)
- **B-Breathing. Establish breathlessness.** After opening the airway establish breathlessness.
  - Turn your head toward the victim's feet with your cheek close over the victim's mouth (3 to 5 seconds).
  - **Look** for a rise and fall in the victim's chest.

- **Listen** for air exchange at the mouth and nose.
- **Feel** for the flow of air.

Sometimes opening and maintaining an open airway is all that is necessary to restore breathing.

- **Provide artificial ventilation**.

  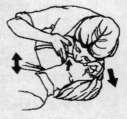

  - If the victim is not breathing give two full breaths by mouth-to-mouth, mouth-to-nose, or mouth-to-stoma ventilation.
  - Allow for lung deflation between each of the two ventilations.

- **C-Circulation. Check for pulse.** Check the victim's pulse to determine whether external cardiac compressions are necessary.

  - Maintain an open airway position by holding the forehead of the victim.

  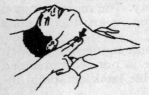

  - Place your fingertips on the victim's windpipe and then slide them towards you until you reach the groove of the neck. Press gently on this area (carotid artery).
  - Check the victim's pulse for at least five seconds but no more than ten.

  - If a pulse is present, continue administering artificial ventilation once every five seconds or twelve times a minute. If not, make arrangements to send for trained medical assistance and begin CPR.

- **Perform cardiac compressions.**
  - Place the victim in a horizontal position on a hard, flat surface.
  - Locate the bottom of the rib cage with the index and middle fingers of your hand closest to patient's feet (*Fig. A*).

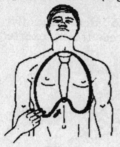 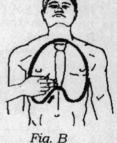

Fig. A   *Fig. B*

- Run your index finger up to or in the notch where the ribs meet the sternum or breast-bone *(Fig. B)*.
- Place your middle finger in notch and index finger on sternum.
- Place the heel of the other hand on the sternum next to the index finger in the notch in the rib cage (below).

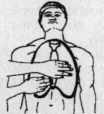 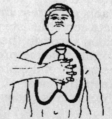

229

- Place the hand used to locate the notch at the rib cage on top and parallel to the hand which is on the sternum.
- Keep the fingers off the chest, by either extending or interlocking them.
- Keep the elbows in a straight and locked position.
  - Position your shoulders directly over the hands so that pressure is exerted straight downward.

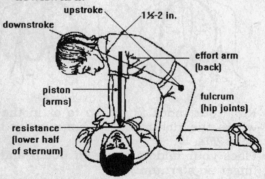

upstroke · 1½-2 in.

downstroke

effort arm (back)

piston (arms)

fulcrum (hip joints)

resistance (lower half of sternum)

- Exert enough downward pressure to depress the sternum of an adult one and one-half to two inches.
- Each compression should squeeze the heart between the sternum and spine to pump blood through the body.
- Totally release pressure in order to allow the heart to refill completely with blood.
- Keep the heel of your hand in contact with the victim's chest at all times.

- Make compressions down and up in a smooth manner.
- Perform fifteen cardiac compressions at a rate of eighty to one hundred per minute, counting "one and, two and, three and," .... to fifteen.
- Use the head-tilt/chin-lift maneuver and give two full breaths (artificial ventilation).
- Repeat cycle four times (fifteen compressions and two ventilations).
- After the fourth cycle, recheck the carotid pulse in the neck for a heartbeat (five to ten seconds).
- If breathing and heartbeat are absent, resume CPR (fifteen compressions and two ventilations).
- Stop and check for heartbeat every few minutes thereafter.
- Never interrupt CPR for more than five seconds except to check the carotid pulse or to move the victim.

Child Resuscitation

Some procedures and rates differ when the victim is a child. Between one and eight years of age, the victim is considered a child. The size of the victim can also be an important factor. A very small nine-year-old victim may have to be treated as a child. Use the following procedures when giving CPR to a child:

- Establish unresponsiveness by the shake and shout method.
- Open the airway using the head-tilt/chin-lift method.
- Establish breathlessness (three to five seconds).
- If the victim is not breathing, give two breaths.
- Check the carotid pulse for at least five seconds.

- Perform cardiac compressions.
  - Place the victim in a horizontal position on a hard, flat surface.
  - Use the index and middle fingers of your hand closest to the patient's feet to locate the bottom of the rib cage.
  - Place your middle finger in notch and index finger on sternum.
  - The heel of the other hand is placed on the sternum next to the index finger in the notch in the rib cage.
  - The fingers must be kept off the chest by extending them.
  - Elbow is kept straight by locking it.
  - The shoulders of the rescuer are brought directly over the hand so that pressure is exerted straight downward.
  - Exert enough pressure downward with one hand to depress the sternum of the child one to one and one-half inches.
  - Compress at a rate of eighty to one hundred times per minute. Ventilate after every five compressions.

Infant Resuscitation

If the victim is younger than one year, it is considered an infant and the following procedures apply:

- Establish unresponsiveness by the shake and shout method.
- Open the airway; take care not to overextend the neck.
- Establish breathlessness (three to five seconds).

232

- Cover the infant's mouth and nose to get an airtight seal.
- Puff cheeks, using the air in the mouth to give two quick ventilations.
- Check the brachial pulse for five seconds.
- To locate the brachial pulse:
  - Place the tips of your index and middle fingers on the inner side of the upper arm.
  - Press slightly on the arm at the groove in the muscle.
- If heartbeat is absent, begin CPR at once:
  - Place the index finger just under an imaginary line between the nipples on the infant's chest. Using the middle and ring fingers, compress chest one-half to one inch.
  - Compress at the rate of at least one hundred times per minute.
  - Ventilate after every five compressions.

Transporting the Victim

Do not interrupt CPR for more than five seconds unless absolutely necessary. When the victim must be moved for safety or transportation reasons, **do not** interrupt CPR for more than thirty seconds.

Termination of CPR

Under normal circumstances CPR may be terminated under one of four conditions:

- The victim is revived
- Another person trained in CPR relieves you
- The person performing CPR becomes exhausted and cannot continue
- A doctor pronounces the victim dead

Controlling Bleeding

Hemorrhaging or Bleeding

Hemorrhaging or bleeding is the escape of blood from an artery, vein, or capillary.

Bleeding from an Artery

Arterial bleeding is characterized by bright red blood that spurts from a wound. The blood in the arteries is pumped directly from the heart, and spurts at each contraction. Having received a fresh supply of oxygen, the blood is bright red.

Bleeding from a Vein

When dark red blood flows from a wound in a steady stream, a vein has been cut. The blood, having given up its oxygen and received carbon dioxide and waste products in return is dark red.

Bleeding from Capillaries

Blood from cut capillaries oozes. There is usually no cause for alarm as relatively little blood is lost. Usually direct pressure with a compress applied over the wound will cause the formation of a clot. When large skin surface is involved, the threat of infection may be more serious than the loss of blood.

"Bleeders"

There are some conditions, such as hemophilia, or those caused by a side affect of medication, etc. that do not allow normal clotting to occur. Some persons may be in danger of bleeding to death even from the slightest wounds. This free bleeding may be internal as well as external, a condition that warrants close observation for shock. In addition to applying compress bandages or gauze, rush the person to the nearest hospital where medical treatment can be quickly administered.

Methods of Controlling Bleeding

Most bleeding can be easily controlled. External bleeding can usually be suppressed by applying direct pressure to the open wound. Direct pressure permits normal blood clotting to occur.

In cases of severe bleeding, the first aider may be upset by the appearance of the wound and the emotional state of the victim. Remember that a small amount of blood emerging from a wound spreads and appears as a lot of blood. It is important for the first aider to keep calm, keep the victim calm and do what is necessary to relieve the situation.

When it is necessary to control bleeding, use the following methods:

- Direct pressure with sterile bandage, if available
- Elevation
- Pressure points
- Direct Pressure
- Tourniquet, if necessary **(as a last resort only)**

Direct Pressure

The best all around method of controlling bleeding is to apply pressure directly to the wound. This is best done by placing gauze or the cleanest material available against the bleeding point and applying firm pressure with the hand until a cover bandage can be applied. The cover bandage knot should be tied over the wound unless otherwise indicated. The bandage supplies direct pressure and should not be removed until the victim is examined by a physician. When air splints or pressure bandages are available, they may be used over the heavy layer of gauze to supply direct pressure.

Bleeding that continues after the bandage is in place indicates that not enough pressure has been applied. In such cases, **do not remove the original dressing**. Use the hand to put more pressure on the wound over the bandage, or apply a second bandage. Either method should control the bleeding.

In severe bleeding, if gauze or other suitable material is not available, the bare hand should be used to apply direct pressure immediately. This will control most bleeding.

Elevation

Elevating the bleeding part of the body above the level of the heart will slow the flow of blood and speed clotting. For example, bleeding from a cut on the hand or arm will be slowed by raising the arm over the head. In the case of a foot wound, the victim should lie down with the leg propped up.

Use elevation with direct pressure when there are no fractures or fractures have been splinted and it will cause no pain or aggravation to the injury.

Pressure Points

Arterial bleeding can be controlled by applying pressure with the finger at *pressure points*. Pressure points are places over a bone where arteries are close to the skin. Pressing the artery against the underlying bone can control the flow of blood to the injury. There are twenty-six pressure points on the body, thirteen on each side, situated along main arteries. (See illustration.)

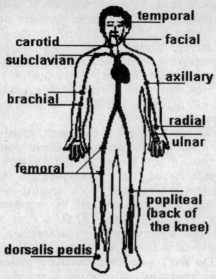

temporal

carotid

facial

subclavian

axillary

brachial

radial

ulnar

femoral

popliteal
(back of
the knee)

dorsalis pedis

In cases of severe bleeding where direct pressure is not adequate to control the bleeding, digital pressure must be used. **Use pressure points with caution**, as indirect pressure may cause damage to the limb as a result of an inadequate flow of blood. When the use of indirect pressure at a pressure point is necessary, **do not** substitute indirect pressure for direct pressure on the wound; use both direct and indirect pressure. Hold the pressure point only as long as necessary to stop the bleeding. Indirect pressure should be reapplied if bleeding recurs.

The *temporal pressure point*, located slightly above

237

and to the side of the eye, is used to control arterial bleeding from a scalp or head wound. It is important that this point be used for brief periods only; as it can cut off blood to the brain and cause damage if held over thirty seconds.

The *facial pressure point* will help slow the flow of blood from a cut on the face. It should be used only for a minute or two. The pressure point is located in the "notch" along the lower edge of the bony structure of the jaw.

When there is bleeding from the neck, locate the trachea at the midline of the neck. Slide your fingers toward the site of the bleeding in the neck and feel for the pulsations of the carotid artery. Place your fingers over the artery, with your thumb behind the patient's neck. Apply pressure by squeezing your fingers toward your thumb. This action will compress the carotid artery against the trachea.

There are few occasions for using the *carotid pressure point*. **Do NOT use this method unless it is a part of your training.** If profuse bleeding from the neck is not controlled by direct pressure, you may have to use this technique. **NEVER apply pressure to both sides of the neck at the same time.** Take great care not to apply heavy pressure to the trachea. Stay alert because the patient may become faint or unconscious. Assume that the cervical spine has been injured and take all necessary steps to avoid excessive movement of the patient's head, neck, and back while you control profuse bleeding. **CAUTION: Maintain pressure for only a few seconds without releasing, since you are shutting off a large supply of oxygenated blood to the brain.**

The *subclavian pressure point* is located deep behind the collar bone in the "sink" of the shoulder. To reach it, you must push your thumb through the thick layer of muscle at the top of the shoulder and press the artery against the collar bone. It should be used only in extreme cases, such as amputation of the arm.

For wounds just above the elbow, the *axillary pressure point* is effective. Here, the artery just under the upper arm is pressed against the bone from underneath.

One of the most effective and most used pressure points for cuts on the lower arm is the *brachial point* at the elbow. Locate this pressure point in a groove on the inside of the arm and the elbow. To apply pressure, grasp the middle of the victim's arm with the thumb on the outside of the arm and the fingers on the inside. Press the fingers toward the thumb. Use the flat inside surface of the fingers, not the fingertips. This inward pressure closes the artery by pressing it against the arm bone.

The *radial pressure point* is located on the forearm close to the wrist on the thumb side of the hand and the *ulnar pressure point* is located on the little finger side of the wrist. The radial pressure point may be used for controlling bleeding at the wrist. Both pressure points must be used at the same time to control bleeding of the hand.

The *femoral artery* is often used to control severe bleeding from a wound on the lower extremity and the amputation of the leg. The pressure point is located on the front, center part of the crease in the groin area. This is where the artery crosses the pelvic basin on the way into the lower extremity. To apply pressure, position the victim flat on his or her back, if possible. Place the heel of one hand directly on the pressure point and apply the small amount of pressure needed to close the artery. If bleeding is not controlled, it may be necessary to press directly over the artery with the flat surface of the fingertips and apply additional pressure on the fingertips with the heel of the other hand.

The *popliteal pressure point* at the back of the knee is the most effective point for controlling bleeding from a wound on the leg. The artery passes close to the surface of the skin, over the large bones in the knee joint.

The *dorsalis pedis pressure point* controls the bleeding in the lower foot and toes. It is found on the top of the foot.

Tourniquet

A tourniquet is a device used to control severe bleeding. **It is used as an absolute last resort after all other methods have failed. First aiders should thoroughly understand the dangers and limitations of its use.**

A tourniquet should normally be used only for life-threatening hemorrhage that cannot be controlled by other means. A tourniquet may be dangerous. Improper use of a tourniquet by inexperienced, untrained persons may cause tissue injury or even death. Use a tourniquet when there is a loss of a limb or to completely shut off the entire blood supply to a limb. The pressure device itself often cuts into or injures the skin and underlying tissue. it is only required when large arteries are severed, in cases of partial or complete severance of a limb, and when bleeding is uncontrollable.

The standard tourniquet usually is a piece of web belting about thirty-six inches long, with a buckle or small device to hold it tightly in place when applied. A tourniquet can be improvised from a strap, belt, suspender, handkerchief, towel, necktie, cloth, or other suitable material. An improvised tourniquet should be at least two inches wide to distribute pressure over tissues. **NEVER use wire, cord, or anything that will cut into the flesh.** A cravat bandage may be used as a tourniquet.

The procedure for application of a tourniquet is as follows:

- While the proper pressure point is being held to temporarily control the bleeding, place the tourniquet between the heart and wound, with sufficient uninjured flesh between the wound and tourniquet.
- In using an improvised tourniquet, wrap the material tightly around the limb twice and tie in a half knot on the upper surface of the limb.
- Place a short stick or similar sturdy object at the half knot and tie a full knot.
- Twist the stick to tighten the tourniquet **only until the bleeding stops**.
- Secure the stick in place with the base ends of the tourniquet, another strip of cloth or suitable material.

Precautions:
- **Do not shield a tourniquet from view.**

- Make a written note of the tourniquet's location and the time it was applied and attach the note to the victim's clothing. Alternatively, make a "T" on the victim's forehead.
- Get the victim to a medical facility as soon as possible.
- Once the tourniquet is tightened, it should not be loosened except by or on the advice of a doctor. The loosening of a tourniquet may dislodge clots and result in sufficient loss of blood to cause severe shock and death.

Internal Bleeding

Internal bleeding in the chest or abdominal cavities usually results from a hard blow or certain fractures. Internal bleeding is usually not visible, but it can be very serious, even fatal. internal bleeding may be determined by any or all of the following signs and symptoms:

- Pain, tenderness, swelling, or discoloration where injury is suspected
- Abdominal rigidity or muscle spasms
- Bleeding from mouth, rectum, or other natural body openings
- Showing symptoms of shock:
  - Dizziness, without other symptoms - dizziness when going from lying to standing may be the only early sign of internal bleeding
  - Cold and clammy skin
  - Eyes dull, vision clouded, and pupils enlarged Weak and rapid pulse
  - Nausea and vomiting
  - Shallow and rapid breathing

- Thirst
- Weak and helpless feeling

Emergency care for internal bleeding requires securing and maintaining an open airway, and treating for shock. **Never give the victim anything by mouth.** Transport anyone suspected of having any internal bleeding to professional medical help as quickly and safely as possible. Keep an injured person on his or her side when blood or vomit is coming from the mouth. Place the victim with chest injuries on the injured side if no spinal injuries are suspected. Transport the victim gently.

Nosebleeds

Nosebleeds are more often annoying than life threatening. They are more common during cold weather, when heated air dries out the nasal passages.

First aid for nosebleeds is simple:

- Keep the victim quietly seated, leaning forward if possible.
- Gently pinch the nostrils closed.
- Apply cold compresses to the victim's nose and face.
- If the person is conscious, it may be helpful to apply pressure beneath the nostril above the lip.
- Instruct victim not to blow his or her nose for several hours after bleeding has stopped or clots could be dislodged and start the bleeding again.

Nosebleeds that cannot be controlled through these measures may signal a more severe condition, such as high blood pressure. The victim should see a physician. Anyone suffering a nosebleed after injury should be examined for possible facial fractures.

If a fractured skull is suspected as the cause of a nosebleed, **do not** attempt to stop the bleeding. To do so might increase the pressure on the brain. Treat the victim for a fractured skull.

Shock

Medically, *shock* is the term used to describe the effects of inadequate circulation of the blood throughout the body. Shock may result from a variety of causes and can cause irreversible harm.

The collapse of the cardiovascular system may be caused by any of three conditions:

- Blood is lost.
- Vessels dilate and there is insufficient blood to fill them.
- The heart fails to act properly as a pump and circulate the blood.

No matter what the reason for the collapse, the results are the same: an insufficient blood flow to provide adequate nourishment and oxygen to all parts of the body. The body process may slow down, reducing circulation and, without nourishment, organs begin to die, especially the brain.

Symptoms of Shock

The signs and symptoms of shock are both physical and emotional. Shock may be determined by any or all of the following conditions:

- Dazed look
- Paleness in light skinned individuals and ashen or grayish color in dark skinned individuals
- Nausea and vomiting

- Thirst
- Weak, rapid pulse
- Cold, clammy skin
- Shallow, irregular, labored breathing
- Pupils dilated
- Eyes dull and lackluster
- Cyanosis, or a bluish tinge to the skin, in the late stages of shock

Some of the reactions known to take place within the body in cases of shock bear directly on the symptoms presented. The most important reaction that occurs in shock is a decided drop in normal blood flow.

The brain suffers from this decreased blood supply and does not function normally; the victim's powers of reasoning, thinking, and expression are dulled. The victim may exhibit the following:

- Weak and helpless feeling
- Anxiety
- Disorientation or confusion
- Unconsciousness, in the late stages of shock

First Aid Treatment for shock

While life threatening, shock is a serious condition which is reversible if recognized quickly and treated effectively. Always maintain an open airway and en-sure adequate breathing; control any bleeding.

First aid for the victim of physical shock is as fol-lows:

- Keep the victim lying down, if possible. Make sure that the head is at least level with the body. Elevate the lower extremities if the injury will not be aggravated and there are no head or abdominal injuries. It may be necessary to raise the head and shoulders if a person is suffering from a head injury, sunstroke, heart attack, stroke, or shortness of breath due to a chest or throat injury. However, it should be noted that if an accident was severe enough to produce a head injury there may also be spinal damage. If in doubt, keep the victim flat.

- Provide the victim with plenty of fresh air.
- Loosen any tight clothing (neck, chest, and waist) in order to make breathing and circulation easier.
- Handle the victim as gently as possible and minimize movement.
- Keep the victim warm and dry by wrapping in blankets, clothing or other available material. These coverings should be placed under as well as over the victim to reduce the loss of body heat. Keep the victim warm enough to be comfortable. The objective is to maintain as near normal body temperature as possible—not to add heat.
- **Do not** give the victim anything by mouth.
- The victim's emotional well-being is just as important as his or her physical well-being. Keep calm and reassure the victim. Never talk to the victim about his or her injuries. Keep onlookers away from the victim as their conversation regarding the victim's injuries may be upsetting.

Anaphylactic Shock

Various technical terms describe different types of shock. At least one of these, anaphylactic shock, is given special emphasis because it is a life-threatening emergency which requires rapid treatment.

Anaphylactic shock is a sensitivity reaction. It occurs when a person contacts something to which he or she is extremely allergic. People who are subject to anaphylactic shock should carry emergency medical identification at all times.

A person can contact substances that can cause anaphylactic shock by eating fish or shellfish, berries, or oral drugs such as penicillin. Insect stings (yellow jackets, wasps, hornets, etc.) or injected drugs can cause a violent reaction, as well as inhaled substances such as dust or pollen.

Sensitivity reactions can occur within a few seconds after contact with the substance. Death can result within minutes of contact; therefore, it is important that the first aider recognize the signs and symptoms of anaphylactic shock:

- Itching or burning skin
- Hives covering a large area
- Swelling of the tongue and face
- Severe difficulty in breathing
- Tightening or pain in the chest
- Weak pulse
- Dizziness
- Convulsion
- Coma

Anaphylactic shock is an emergency that requires medication to counteract the allergic reaction. If the victim carries any medication to counteract the allergy, help the victim take the medicine.

Arrange for transportation to a medical facility as

quickly as possible because anaphylactic shock can be fatal in less than fifteen minutes. Notify the hospital as to what caused the reaction, if known. Maintain an open airway. If necessary, provide artificial ventilation and CPR and treat for physical shock.

Fainting

Fainting is a temporary loss of consciousness due to an inadequate supply of oxygen to the brain and is a mild form of shock. Fainting may be caused by the sight of blood, exhaustion, weakness, heat, or strong emotions such as fright, joy, etc.

The signs and symptoms of fainting may be any or all of the following:

- The victim may feel weak and dizzy, and may see spots.
- The face becomes pale and the lips blue in both light and dark skinned people.
- The forehead is covered with cold perspiration.
- The pulse is rapid and weak.
- The breathing is shallow.

The first aid for fainting is as follows:

- If a person feels faint, the initial response might be sitting with the head between the knees.
- Have the victim lie down with the head lower than the feet.
- If the victim is unconscious for any length of time, something may be seriously wrong. Arrange for transportation to a medical facility.
- Treat the victim for physical shock.
- Maintain an open airway.
- **Do not** give stimulants.

Treating Wounds

Open Wounds

An *open wound* refers to any break in the skin. The skin affords protection from most bacteria or germs; however, germs may enter through even a small break in the skin, and an infection may develop.

Breaks in the skin range from pin punctures or scratches to extensive cuts, tears, or gashes. An open wound may be the only surface evidence of a more serious injury such as a fracture, particularly in the case of head injuries involving fracture of the skull. In first aid, open wounds are divided into six classifications: Abrasions, amputations, avulsions, incisions, lacerations, and punctures.

Abrasions

Abrasions are caused by rubbing or scraping. These wounds are seldom deep, but a portion of the skin has been damaged, leaving a raw surface with minor bleeding. The bleeding in most abrasions is from the capillaries. Abrasions are easily infected due to the top layer of skin being removed leaving the underlying skin exposed.

Amputations

An amputation involves the extremities. When an amputation occurs, the fingers, toes, hands, feet, or limbs are completely cut through or torn off which causes jagged skin and exposed bone. Bleeding may be excessive or the force that amputates a limb may close off torn vessels and limit the bleeding. A clean cut amputation seals off vessels and minimizes bleeding. A torn amputation usually bleeds heavily.

Avulsions

An avulsion is an injury that tears an entire piece of skin and tissue loose or leaves it hanging as a flap. This type of wound usually results when tissue is forcibly separated or torn from the victim's body. There is great danger of infection and bleeding. Body parts that have been wholly or partly torn off may sometimes be successfully reattached by a surgeon.

Incisions

Wounds produced by a sharp cutting edge, such as a knife or razor, are referred to as incised wounds. The edges of such wounds are smooth without tearing or bruising. If such a wound is deep, large blood vessels and nerves may be severed. Incised wounds bleed freely, and are often difficult to control.

Lacerations

Lacerated wounds are those with rough or jagged edges. The flesh has been torn or mashed by blunt instruments, machinery, or rough edges such as a jagged piece of metal.

Because the blood vessels are torn or mashed, these wounds may not bleed as freely as incised wounds. The ragged and torn tissues, with the foreign matter that is often forced or ground into the wound make it difficult to determine the extent of the damage. The danger of infection is great in lacerations.

Punctures

Puncture wounds are produced by pointed objects such as needles, splinters, nails, or pieces of wire that pass through the skin and damage tissue in their path. The small number of blood vessels cut sometimes prevents free bleeding. The danger of infection in puncture wounds is great due to this poor drainage.

There are two types of puncture wounds:

- A *penetrating puncture wound* causes injured tissues and blood vessels whether it is shallow or deep.
- A *perforating puncture wound* has an entrance and exit wound. The object causing the injury passes through the body and out to create an exit wound which in many cases is more serious than the entrance wound.

First Aid for Open Wounds

The chief duties of a first aider in caring for open wounds are to stop bleeding and to prevent germs from entering the wound. If germs do not enter, there will be much less chance of infection and the wound will heal quickly.

- Carefully cut or tear the clothing so that the injury may be seen.
- If loose foreign particles are around the wound, wipe them away with clean material. **Always wipe away from the wound, not toward it**.
- **Do not** attempt to remove an object impaled in the wound. Serious bleeding and other damage may occur if the object is removed. Stabilize the object with a bulky dressing.
- **Do not** touch the wound with your hands, clothing, or anything that is not clean, if possible.
- Place a sterile bandage compress or gauze, when available, over the wound and tie in place.

- Dressings should be wide enough to completely cover the wound and the area around it.
- Protect compresses, or gauze dressings with a cover bandage made from a cravat or triangular bandage. Place outer dressings on all open wounds except for wounds of the eye, nose, chin, finger and toe, or compound fractures of the hand and foot when splints are applied. Either use a cravat bandage or triangular bandage to cover the entire dressing.
- Unless otherwise specified, tie the knots of the bandage compress and outer dressing over the wound on top of the compress pad to help in checking the bleeding. However, when an open fracture is involved, tie away from wound.
- Keep victim quiet and lying still. Any movement will increase circulation which could restart bleeding.
- Reassure the victim to ease emotional reaction.
- Treat for shock.

First Aid Dressings and Bandages

First aid materials for dressings and bandages include:

- Bandage compress
- Gauze
- Roller bandage
- Adhesive compress
- Triangular bandage
- Cravat bandage

Bandage Compress

A bandage compress is a special dressing intended

to cover open wounds. It consists of a pad made of several thicknesses of gauze attached to the middle of a strip of gauze. Pad sizes range from one to four inches. Bandage compresses usually come folded so that the gauze pad can be applied directly to the open wound with virtually no exposure to the air or fingers. The strip of gauze at either side of the gauze pad is folded back so that it can be opened and the bandage compress tied in place with no disturbance of the sterile pad. The gauze of a bandage compress may be extended to twice its normal size by opening up folded gauze. Unless otherwise specified, all bandage compresses and all gauze dressings should be covered with an open triangular cravat or roller bandage.

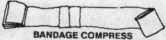

BANDAGE COMPRESS

Gauze

Gauze is used in several ways to apply first aid dressings. Plain gauze may be used in place of a bandage compress to cover large wounds and wounds of the trunk. Plain gauze of various sizes is supplied in packets. In cases of profuse bleeding or where bulk is required to stabilize embedded objects, use several layers of gauze. Care should be taken not to touch the portion of the gauze that is to be placed in contact with the wound.

Gauze Roller Bandage

The gauze roller bandage is a self-adhering form-fitting bandage. It can be made secure with several snug overlapping wraps then tied in place.

Adhesive Compress

An adhesive compress is a self-adhering bandage that has gauze to cover the wound and a sticky backing which holds to the victim's skin.

Triangular Bandage

A standard triangular bandage is made from a piece of cloth approximately forty inches square by folding the square diagonally and cutting along the fold. It is easily applied and can be handled so that the part to be applied over wound or burn dressings will not be soiled.

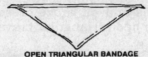

OPEN TRIANGULAR BANDAGE

A triangular bandage does not tend to slip off once it is correctly applied. It is usually made from unbleached cotton cloth, although any kind of cloth will do. In emergencies, a triangular bandage can be improvised from a clean handkerchief, a clean piece of shirt, etc.

The triangular bandage is also used to make improvised tourniquets, to support fractures and dislocations, to apply splints, and to form slings. If a regular-size bandage is found to be too short when a dressing is applied, it can be lengthened by tying another bandage to one end.

Cravat Bandages

A triangular bandage may be used open or folded. When folded, it is known as a cravat. A cravat bandage is prepared as follows:

- Make a one inch fold along the base of the triangular bandage.
- Bring the point (apex) to the center of the folded base, placing the point underneath the fold, to make a *wide cravat* bandage.
- A *medium cravat* is made by folding lengthwise along a line midway between the base and the new top of the bandage, in effect, folding the wide cravat bandage in half lengthwise.
- A *narrow cravat* is made by repeating the folding.

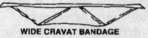

WIDE CRAVAT BANDAGE

This method has the advantage that all bandages can be folded to a uniform width, or the width may be varied to suit the purpose for which it is to be used. To complete a dressing, the ends of the bandage are tied securely.

Square Knot

Unless otherwise specified, all knots or ties mentioned in this manual should be tied in a square knot.

To tie a square knot, take an end of the bandage in each hand, pass the end in the right hand over and around the end in the left and tie a single knot. Then pass the end now in the left hand over the end in the right hand, and complete the knot. Each loose end, after the second knot is tied, will be doubled back and lying against itself with the other end wrapped around it. The rule to remember in tying a square knot is right over left, then left over right.

Slings

Slings are used to support injuries of the shoulder, upper extremities or ribs. In an emergency they may be improvised from belts, neckties, scarves, or similar articles. Bandages should be used if available.

Triangular Bandage Sling

Tie a triangular bandage sling as follows:

- Place one end of the base of an open triangular bandage over the shoulder on the injured side.
- Allow the bandage to hang down in front of the chest so that the apex, or point, will be behind the elbow of the injured arm.
- Bend the arm at the elbow with hand slightly elevated (four to five inches).
- Bring the forearm across the chest and over the bandage.
- Carry the lower end of the bandage over the shoulder on the uninjured side and tie at uninjured side of the neck, being sure the knot is at the side of the neck.
- Twist the apex of the bandage, and tuck it in at the elbow.

The hand should be supported with the fingertips exposed, whenever possible, to permit detection of interference with circulation.

Cravat Bandage Sling

Tie a cravat bandage sling as follows:

- Place one end over the shoulder on the injured side.
- Allow the bandage to hang down in front of the chest.

- Bend the arm at the elbow with hand slightly elevated four to five inches.
- Bring the forearm across the chest and over the bandage.
- Carry the lower end of the bandage over the injured arm to the shoulder on the uninjured side and tie at uninjured side of neck.

Basket Sling

A useful sling for transporting or handling a victim with a suspected neck injury or an unconscious victim whose arms may create difficulties, can be made with an open triangular bandage as follows:

- Place an open triangular bandage across the chest with the apex down.
- Fold the arms over one another on the bandage. Bring the ends of the base together and tie.
- Cross the apex over the folded arms and tie to the knotted ends of the base.

Principles of Bandaging

- Bandage wounds snugly, but not too tightly. Too tight a bandage may damage surrounding tissue or interfere with the blood supply, especially if swelling occurs. A bandage tied too loosely may slip off the wound.
- In bandaging the arms or the legs, leave the tips of the fingers or toes uncovered where possible to detect any interference with circulation.
- If the victim complains that the bandage is too tight, loosen it to make it comfortable, but snug. Unless otherwise specified, all knots should be tied over open wounds to help control bleeding.

• If bandages become saturated with blood, apply additional bandages or dressings. **Do not** remove original dressing.

Dressings for Wounds

The following dressings are recommended for covering wounds.

Scalp, Temple, Ear, or Face

To dress an open wound for the scalp, temple, ear, or face, proceed as follows:

• Apply the pad of a bandage compress over the wound.
• Carry one end under the chin, and the other over the top of the head.
• Cross at the temple in front of the ear on the side opposite the injury (illustration below, left).
• Bring one end around the front of the head and the other end low around the back of the head.
• Tie on or near the compress pad.
• Cover the compress with a cravat bandage applied in the same manner.

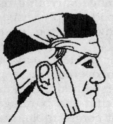 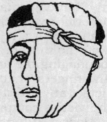

If the wound is on the cheek or the front of the face, cross the bandage compress and cravat bandage behind the ear, on the side opposite the injury; bring the ends around the forehead and back of the head, and tie (illustration above, right).

Extensive Wounds of the Scalp

A wound or wounds involving a large area of the scalp may be dressed by covering the injury with a piece of gauze or a large bandage compress.

- Apply the pad of a sterile compress to the wound.
- Carry one end under the chin and the other end over the top of the head.
- Cross the ends at the temple.
- Carry one end around the forehead.
- Pass the other end around the back of the head and tie on the opposite side of the face.
- Next apply a triangular bandage over the head with the base snugly across the forehead, just above the eyebrows and the apex of the bandage at the back of the neck.
- Bring the two ends of the bandage around the head just above the ears.
- Cross under the bony prominence on the back of the head.
- Return the ends to the middle of the forehead.
- Tie just above the eyebrows.
- Fold up the apex and tuck it in snugly over the crossed ends at the back of the head.

When gauze is used, take care to keep it in place while the cover bandage is being applied.

Forehead or Back of Head

To dress an open wound of the forehead or back of the head, proceed as follows:

- Apply the pad of a sterile bandage compress over the injury.
- Hold the compress in place by passing the ends of the compress around the head above the ears, and tying over the compress pad.
- Apply the center of a cravat bandage over the pad, take the ends around the head, cross them, and tie over the compress pad.

Eye Injuries

Objects embedded in the eye should be removed only by a doctor. Such objects must be protected from accidental movement or removal until the victim receives medical attention.

- Tell the victim that both eyes must be bandaged to protect the injured eye.
- Encircle the eye with a gauze dressing or other suitable material.
- Position a cup or cone over the embedded object. The object should not touch the top or sides of the cup. It may be necessary to make a hole in the bottom of the cup if the object is longer than the cup.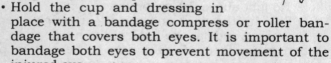
- Hold the cup and dressing in place with a bandage compress or roller bandage that covers both eyes. It is important to bandage both eyes to prevent movement of the injured eye.
- Never leave the victim alone, as the victim may panic with both eyes covered. Keep in hand contact so the victim will always know someone is there.

- Stabilize the head with sand bags or large pads and always transport the victim on his or her back.
- Ensure that the victim does not tamper with the dressing or embedded object.

This procedure should also be used for lacerations and other injuries to the eyeball.

After a serious injury, the eyeball may be knocked out of the socket. No attempt should be made to put the eye back into the socket. The eye should be covered with a moist dressing and a protective cup without applying pressure to the eye. A bandage compress or roller bandage that covers both eyes should be applied. Transport the victim face up with the head immobilized.

For all injuries to and around the upper or lower lid of the eye, use a sterile bandage compress as follows:

- Place the center of a bandage compress over the injured eye.
- Carry the end on the injured side below the ear to the back of the head.
- Carry the other end above the ear on the opposite side.
- Tie toward the injured side below the bony prominence on the back of the head.
- Bring both ends over the top of the head, passing the longer end under the dressing at the temple on the uninjured side.
- Slide it in front of the uninjured eye and pull it tightly enough to raise the dressing above the uninjured eye.
- Tie to the other end on top of the head.

Nose

To bandage a wound to the nose, proceed as follows:
- Split the tails of a bandage compress.
- Apply the pad of the compress to the wound.
- Pass the top tails, one to each side of the head below the ears and tie at the back of the neck.
- Pass the bottom tails, one to each side of the head above the ears and tie at the back of the head.

Chin

In order to tie a bandage for a wound on the chin, proceed as follows:
- Split the tails of a bandage compress. Apply the pad of the compress to the wound.
- Pass the top tails, one to each side of the neck, below the ears and tie at the back of the neck.
- Pass the bottom tails, one to each side of the head in front of the ears and tie at the top of the head.

Neck or Throat

To bandage a wound on the neck or throat, proceed as follows:
- Apply the pad of a sterile bandage compress to the wound.
- Pass the ends around the neck, and tie over the wound.
- Place the center of cravat bandage over the compress.
- Pass the ends of the cravat bandage around the neck, cross them, bring them around the neck again, and tie loosely.
- Use hand pressure over the wound for control of

excessive bleeding.

Shoulder

In order to tie a bandage for a wound of the shoulder, proceed as follows:

- Apply the pad of a bandage compress over the wound. Bring the ends under the armpit.
- Cross, carry to the top of the compress, cross, carry one end across the chest and one end across the back, and tie in the opposite armpit over a pad.
- Place the apex of a triangular bandage high up on the shoulder. Place the base, along which a hem has been folded, below the shoulder on the upper part of the arm, carry the ends around the arm and tie them on the outside.
- To hold the bandage in position, place the center of a cravat bandage under the opposite armpit; carry the ends to the shoulder over the apex of the first bandage; tie a single knot; then fold the apex over and complete the knot.
- Place the forearm in a triangular bandage sling.

Armpit

To dress a wound of the armpit, proceed as follows:

- Apply the pad of a bandage compress over the wound. Lift the arm only high enough to apply compress, as further damage may occur to lacerated nerves which are close to the surface.
- Carry the ends over the shoulder and cross.
- Carry one end across the chest and the other end across the back.
- Tie under the opposite arm over a pad.
  - **If there is severe bleeding**, place a hard

object over the pad of the compress and push it well up into the armpit, holding the pads in place by a cravat bandage.
- Place the center of a cravat bandage over the wound.
- Bring the ends over the shoulder, crossing them; then pass the ends around the chest and back and tie them under the opposite arm. Next bring the arm down and secure it firmly against the chest wall by a cravat bandage passed around the arm and chest. Tie securely on the opposite side over a pad.
- Place the forearm in a triangular sling.

Arm, Forearm, and Wrist

To bandage wounds of the arm, forearm, and wrist, proceed as follows:
- Apply the pad of a sterile bandage compress over the wound.
- Pass the ends several times around the arm and tie them over the pad.
- Place the center of a cravat bandage over the pad.
- Pass the ends around the arm, cross them, continue around the arm and tie over the pad.
- Place the forearm and hand in a triangular sling.

Elbow

To dress a wound of the elbow, proceed as follows:
- Start with joint in a slightly bent position.
- Apply the pad of a bandage compress over the wound.
- Pass the ends of the bandage around the elbow

and carry them around the arm just above the elbow.

- Cross them and carry them around the forearm just below the elbow.
- Tie at a point below the elbow.

Cover with a cravat bandage as follows:

- Place the center of the cravat bandage over the point of the elbow.
- Pass the ends around and cross them above the point of the elbow.
- Carry them around the arm and cross again at the bend of the elbow.
- Carry around the forearm, and tie just below the point of the elbow.
- Immobilize the upper extremity by placing the forearm in a triangular sling.

Palm or Back of Hand

To dress a wound of the palm or back of the hand, proceed as follows:

- Apply the pad of a bandage compress over the wound.
- Pass the ends several times around the hand and wrist.
- Tie over the pad.
- Place the center of a cravat bandage over the pad.
- Cross the ends at the opposite side of the hand.
- Pass one end around the little finger side of the hand.
- Pass the other end between the thumb and forefinger, taking the ends to the wrist.
- Cross the ends and continue around the wrist,

crossing at the back of the wrist.
- Cross again at the inside of the wrist.

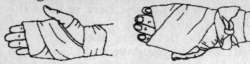

- Tie at the back of the wrist.
- Place the forearm and hand in a triangular bandage sling.

Extensive Wounds of the Hand

Control arterial bleeding of the hand.

To dress extensive wounds of the hand, proceed as follows:

- Apply gauze or a bandage compress over the wound.
- When there are multiple wounds of fingers, separate the fingers with gauze.
- If a bandage compress is used, pass the ends several times around the hand and wrist.
- Tie them over the pad.

Cover the hand with a triangular bandage as follows:

- Place the base on the inner side of the wrist.
- Bring the apex down over the back of the hand.
- Cross the ends (little finger side first) over the back of the hand and wrist.
- Wrap around wrist, ending in tie on back of wrist.
- Bring the apex down over the knot and tuck it under.
- Place the forearm and hand in a triangular bandage sling.
- If there is swelling, elevate and apply ice.

Finger

To dress a wound of the finger, proceed as follows:

- Apply the pad of a small bandage compress over the wound.
- Pass the ends several times around the finger and tie over the pad.
- A small adhesive compress may be used instead of a bandage compress for a wound of the finger or a wound on the end of the finger. A bent finger should be dressed bent and not fully extended.
- If more than one finger is injured, cover with an open triangular bandage as for extensive wounds of the hand.

Chest or Back Between Shoulder Blades

To dress a wound on the chest or back between the shoulder blades, proceed as follows:

- Place the pad of the compress over the wound so that the ends are diagonally across the chest or back.
- Carry one end over the shoulder and under the armpit. Carry the other end under the armpit and over the shoulder. Tie the ends over the compress.

Cover the compress and chest or back with a triangular bandage as follows:

- Place the center of the base at the lower part of the neck.
- Allow the apex to drop down over the chest or back, as appropriate.
- Carry the ends over the shoulders and under the armpits to the center of the chest or back.

- Tie with the apex below the knot.
- Turn the apex up and tuck it over the knot.

Back, Chest, Abdomen, Or Side

To tie a bandage for the back, chest, abdomen, or side, proceed as follows:

- Apply the pad of a sterile bandage compress or sterile gauze over the wound. If a sterile bandage compress is used, take the ends around the body (one end across the back and the other across the abdomen or chest and tie on the side).
- Cover with a proper size cravat bandage by placing the center of the bandage on the side nearest the injury.
- Take the ends across the back and abdomen or chest and tie on the opposite side.

NOTE: If air is being sucked into the lungs through a wound in the chest, cover the wound immediately with a nonporous material, such as plastic wrap, wax paper, or your hand; then dress the wound. Transport the victim to a medical facility as quickly as possible.

Protruding Intestines

To dress a wound in which the victim's intestines are protruding, proceed as follows:

- Place the victim on his or her back with something under the knees to raise them and help relax the abdominal muscles.
- **Do not** try to re-place the intestines; leave the organ on the surface.
- Cover with aluminum foil, plastic wrap, or a moist dressing.

- Cover lightly with an outer dressing. This will help preserve heat.

Lower Abdomen, Back, or Buttocks

To dress a wound of the lower part of the abdomen, the lower part of the back or the buttocks, proceed as follows:

- Apply a pad made from several layers of sterile gauze; in the absence of gauze, the pad of a sterile compress may be placed over the wound and held in place by passing the ends around the body and tying them.
- Cover the gauze or bandage compress with two triangular bandages:
- Tie the apexes in the crotch.
- Bring the base of one bandage up on the abdomen.
- Pass the ends around to the back and tie.
- Pass the ends of the other bandage around to the front and tie.

Groin

To dress a wound of the groin, proceed as follows:

- Apply the pad of a bandage compress over the wound.
- Carry the ends to the hip and cross.
- Carry the ends across to the opposite side of the body and tie.

Cover the compress with two cravat bandages tied together as follows:

- Place the center of one of the cravat bandages over the pad and follow the compress in such a manner as to cover it entirely.
- Continue with the other cravat bandage around

the entire body a second time and tie.

Crotch

To bandage a wound of the crotch, proceed as follows:

- Cover wound with sterile gauze.
- Pass a narrow cravat bandage around the waist and tie in front, leaving the ends to hang free.
- Pass a second cravat bandage under the knot of the first cravat bandage.
- Pass the two ends of the second cravat bandage between the thighs and bring one end around each hip.
- Tie to the ends of the cravat bandage tied around the body.

Hip

To dress a wound of the hip, proceed as follows:

- Split the tails of a bandage compress.
- Place the pad over the wound.
- Pass the top tails around the body.
- Tie over the opposite hip.
- Pass the ends of the bottom tails around thigh and cross on inside of thigh.
- Continue around the thigh, tying on the outside.

Cover with a triangular bandage as follows:

- Place the base of a triangular bandage on the thigh with the apex pointing up; bring the ends of the base around the thigh, and tie.
- Pass a second cravat bandage around the body at the waist and tie a single knot over the apex of the triangular bandage.
- Fold the apex over the knot and complete tying the knot.

Thigh or Leg

To tie a bandage for a wound of the thigh or leg, proceed as follows:

- Apply the pad of a bandage compress over the wound.
- Pass the ends around the injured extremity and tie over the pad.
- Place the center of a cravat bandage over the compress, pass the ends around the injured part, cross them, bring them around again, and tie over the pad.

Knee

To dress a wound of the knee, proceed as follows:

- Apply the pad of a sterile bandage compress over the wound.
- Cross the ends at the back of the knee and return to the front of the knee.
- Tie firmly over the pad, if possible.
- Place the center of a cravat bandage over the pad.
- Bring the ends of the bandage around each side of the leg.
- Cross them at the back of the knee, pull them forward, and tie them above the knee.

Ankle

To dress a wound of the ankle, proceed as follows:

- Apply the pad of a bandage compress to the wound.
- Carry the ends to the top of the instep and cross.
- Carry the ends around the bottom of the foot and cross over the instep again.

- Pass the ends around the ankle and tie over the pad.
- Place the center of a cravat bandage over the compress.
- Carry the ends to the top of the instep, cross.
- Cross the ends under the foot, bring back to the top of the instep and cross.
- Carry the ends around the ankle and tie over the pad.

Foot

To dress a wound of the foot proceed as follows:

- Apply the pad of a bandage compress to the wound.
- Carry the ends around the foot and ankle.
- Tie over the pad.
- Place the center of a cravat bandage over the compress.
- Carry the ends around the foot and ankle, ending in a tie as near the front of the ankle as possible.

Extensive Wounds of Foot or Toes

First, control arterial bleeding of the foot.

To dress extensive wounds of the foot and toes, proceed as follows:

- Apply gauze or the pad of a large bandage compress over the wound and tie it in place.
- Place the base of a triangular bandage on the back of the ankle.
- Bring the apex under the sole of the foot, over the toes, back over the instep, and up the leg to

a point above the ankle in front.

- Pass the end on the little toe side over the instep, then the other end over the instep, and continue around the ankle with both ends and tie in front.
- Bring the apex down over the knot and tuck in under the knot.

Toe

To dress a wound of the toe, proceed as follows:

- Apply the pad of a small bandage compress over the wound.
- Pass the ends around the toe several times and tie over the pad.
- Instead of a bandage compress a small adhesive compress may be used for a wound of the toe or a wound on the end of the toe.
- When there are multiple wounds of the toes, separate the toes with gauze. Cover with a triangular bandage as described for extensive wounds of the foot.

Closed Wounds

Closed wounds are injuries where the skin is not broken, but damage occurs to underlying tissues. These injuries may result in internal bleeding from damage to internal organs, muscles, and other tissues. Closed wounds are classified as follows:

- Bruises
- Ruptures or hernias

Bruises

Bruises are caused by an object striking the body or the body coming into contact with a hard object, for example in a fall or a bump. The skin is not broken, but the soft tissue beneath the skin is damaged. Small blood vessels are ruptured, causing blood to seep into surrounding tissues. This produces swelling. The injured area appears red at first, then darkens to blue or purple. When large blood vessels have been ruptured or large amounts of underlying tissue have been damaged, a lump may develop as a result of the blood collecting within the damaged tissue. This lump is called a hematoma or blood tumor. The symptoms of a bruise are as follows:

- Immediate pain
- Swelling
- Rapid discoloration
- Later, pain or pressure on movement

The first aid for bruises is as follows:

- To limit swelling and reduce pain, apply an ice bag, a cloth wrung out in cold water, or a chemical cold pack.
- Elevate the injured area and place at complete rest.
- Check for fractures and other possible injuries.
- Treat for shock.

Severe bruises should have the care of a doctor.

Ruptures or Hernias

The most common form of rupture or hernia is a protrusion of a portion of an internal organ through the wall of the abdomen. Most ruptures occur in or just above the groin, but they may occur at other places over the abdomen. Ruptures result from a combination of weakness of the tissues and muscular strain.

The symptoms of a rupture are as follows:

- Sharp, stinging pain
- Feeling of something giving away at the site of the rupture
- Swelling
- Possible nausea and vomiting

The first aid for an individual who has suffered a rupture is as follows:

- Place the victim on his or her back with the knees well drawn up.
- Place a blanket or similar padding under the knees.
- Place the center of a cravat under the padding, bring the ends above the knees and tie.
- Place the center of two cravat bandages tied together at the ends on the outside of the thighs and pass the ends around the thighs, cross under the blanket, bring the ends around the legs just above the ankles and tie.
- Never attempt to force the protrusion back into the cavity.
- Place cold application to injured area.
- Cover with a blanket.
- The victim should be transported lying down with the knees drawn up.

Foreign Bodies

Foreign Bodies in the Eye

Foreign bodies such as particles of dirt, dust, or fine pieces of metal may enter the eye and lodge there. If not removed, they can cause discomfort, inflammation and possibly, infection.

Through an increased flow of tears, nature limits the possibility of harm by dislodging many of these substances. **Do not** let the victim rub the eye. Rubbing may scratch the delicate eye tissues or force sharp objects into the tissues. This makes removal of the object difficult. The first aider should not attempt to remove foreign bodies. It is always much safer to send the person to a physician.

To remove a foreign body on the inside of the eyelid, proceed as follows:

- Pull upper eyelid down over the lower eyelashes.
- Lift eyelid and remove object with sterile gauze.

The first aid for a foreign body on the eye that is not on the cornea or imbedded is as follows:

- Flush the eye with clean water, if available, for 15 minutes. If necessary, hold the eyelids apart.
- Often a foreign body lodged under the upper eyelid can be removed by drawing the upper lid down over the lower lid; as the upper lid returns to its normal position, the under surfaces will be drawn over the lashes of the lower lid and the foreign body removed by the wiping action of the eyelashes.
- A foreign body on the surface of the eye may also be removed by grasping the eyelashes of the upper lid and turning the lid over a cotton swab or similar object. The particle may then be carefully removed from the eyelid with the corner of a piece of sterile gauze.

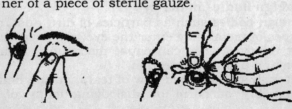

If a foreign body becomes lodged in the eyeball, **do not** attempt to disturb it, as it may be forced deeper into the eye and result in further damage. Place a bandage compress over both eyes. Keep the victim calm and get medical help.

Foreign Bodies in the Ear

Small insects, pieces of rock, or other material may become lodged in the ear. Children sometimes put other objects, such as kernels of corn, peas, buttons or seeds in their ears. Such objects as seeds absorb moisture and swell in the ear, making their removal difficult and often causing inflammation.

The first aid for foreign bodies in the ear is as follows:

- **Do not** insert pins, match sticks, pieces of wire or other objects in the ear to dislodge foreign bodies because this may damage the tissue lining of the ear or perforate the ear drum.
- In the case of insects, turn the victim's head to the side and put several drops of warm olive oil, mineral oil, or baby oil in the ear; then let the oil run out and the drowned insect may come out with it. **Do not** try to flush out objects with water.
- Consult a physician if a foreign body cannot be easily removed.

Foreign Bodies in the Nose

Foreign bodies in the nose usually can be removed without difficulty, but occasionally the services of a physician are required.

The first aid is as follows:

- Induce sneezing by sniffing snuff or pepper, or

tickling the opposite nostril with a feather. This will usually dislodge a foreign body in the nose.

- **Do not** blow the nose violently or with one nostril held shut.
- **Do not** attempt to dislodge the foreign body with a hairpin or similar object. This method may damage tissues of the nasal cavity or push the foreign body into an inaccessible place.

Foreign Bodies in the Stomach

Foreign bodies such as pins coins, nails, and other objects are sometimes swallowed accidentally. Except for pins, nails, or other sharp objects, foreign objects that are swallowed usually cause no great harm.

The first aid for a foreign body in the stomach is as follows:

- **Do not** give anything to induce vomiting or bowel movement.
- Consult a physician immediately.

Burns and Scalds

Classification of Burns

Burns may be classified according to extent and depth of damage as follows:

• First degree Minor	Burned area is painful. Outer skin is reddened. Slight swelling is present.
• Second degree Moderate	Burned area is painful. Underskin is affected. Blisters may form. The area may have a wet, shiny appearance because of exposed tissue.
• Third degree Critical	Insensitive due to the destruction of nerve endings. Skin is destroyed. Muscle tissues and bone underneath may be damaged. The area may be charred, white, or grayish in color.

Burns may also be classified according to cause. The four major types of burns by cause are as follows:

- Chemical
- Thermal
- Electrical
- Radiation

The seriousness of a burn or scald is influenced by the extent of the body surface involved, as well as by the depth to which the tissue has been penetrated. It is generally assumed that where two-thirds of the surface of the body is injured by a second degree burn or scald, death will usually follow, but a much smaller area injured by a third-degree burn can also cause death.

Burns can do more damage than injure the skin. Burns can damage muscles, bones, nerves, and blood vessels. The eyes can be burned beyond repair. The respiratory system structures can be damaged, with possible airway obstruction, respiratory failure, and respiratory arrest. In addition to the physical damage caused by burns, victims also may suffer emotional and psychological problems that could last a lifetime.

Shock is very severe when burns are extensive and may cause death in a few hours.

First Aid for Burns

The first aid given to a burn victim largely depends on the cause of the burn and the degree of severity.

Emergency first aid for burns or scalds should primarily be:

- Exclusion of air from the burned area
- Relief of the pain that immediately follows burns
- Minimizing the onset of shock
- Prevention of infection.

Remove all clothing from the injured area, but cut around any clothing that adheres to the skin and leave it in place. Keep the patient covered, except the injured part, since there is a tendency to chill.

First aid dressings for burns and scalds should be free of grease or oil. The use of greases or oils in the treatment of burns makes it necessary to cleanse the burned or scalded areas with a solvent before medical treatment can begin. This delays the medical treatment and is very painful.

Be careful when dressing burns and scalds. Burned and scalded surfaces are subject to infection the same as open wounds and require the same care to prevent infection. **Do not** break blisters intentionally.

Never permit burned surfaces to be in contact with each other, such as areas between the fingers or toes, the ears and the side of the head, the undersurface of the arm and the chest wall, the folds of the groin, and similar places.

Cover bandages should be loose enough to prevent pressure on burned surfaces. Swelling often takes place after burn dressings have been applied, so check them frequently to see that they are not too tight. Watch for evidence of shock and treat if it is present.

In cases of severe burns, remove the victim to the hospital as quickly as possible. The victim will probably require an anesthetic so that ordinarily nothing should be given by mouth.

In addition to the general principles listed, certain other principles must be followed when giving first aid for specific types of burns.

Chemical Burns of the Eyes

Frequently chemical substances, especially lime, cement, caustic soda, or acids or alkalis from storage batteries get into the eyes. The treatment is to wash the eyes freely with clean water. To do this, have the victim lie down, hold the eyelids open with the fingers and pour the water into the inner corner of the eyes from a pitcher or other container. Use plenty of water and wash the eyes thoroughly, being sure the water actually flows across the eyes. **Do not** put neutralizing solution in the eyes. Cover both eyes with moistened sterile gauze pads and secure in place. Chemical burns of the eyes should receive the attention of an eye specialist as soon as possible.

Chemical Burns

General first aid for chemical burns is as follows:

- Remove all clothing containing the chemical agent.
- **Do not** use any neutralizing solution, unless recommended by a physician.
- Irrigate with water for at least 15 minutes, use potable water if possible.
- Treat for shock.
- Transport to a medical facility.

First aid for dry chemical (alkali) burns is an exception to the general first aid for chemical burns because mixing water with dry alkali creates a corrosive substance. The dry alkali should be brushed from the skin and water should then be used in very large amounts.

Minor Thermal Burns

General first aid for minor thermal burns is as follows:

- Use cool, moist applications of gauze or bandage material to minimize blistering.
- Treat for physical shock.

If the victim has thermal burns on the eyelids, apply moist, sterile gauze pads to both eyes and secure in place.

Moderate or Critical Thermal Burns

General first aid for more serious thermal burns is as follows:

- **Do not** use cold applications on extensive burns; cold could cause chilling.
- Cover the burn with a clean, dry dressing.
- Treat for shock.
- Transport to a medical facility.

Electrical Burns

General first aid for electrical burns is as follows:

- Conduct a primary survey, as cardiac and respiratory arrest can occur in cases of electrical burns.
- Check for points of entry and exit of current.
- Cover burned surface with a clean dressing.
- Splint all fractures. (Violent muscle contractions caused by the electricity may result in fractures.)
- Treat for physical shock.
- Transport to a medical facility.

Respiratory failure and cardiac arrest are the major problems caused by electrical shock and **not** the burn. Monitor pulse and breathing while preparing victim for transportation.

Radiation Burns

Radiation presents a hazard to the rescuer as well as the victim. A rescuer who must enter a radioactive area should stay for as short a time as possible. Radiation is undetectable by the human senses and the rescuer, while attempting to aid the victim, may receive a fatal dose of radiation without realizing it. Notify experts immediately of possible radioactive contamination.

Burns of the Face, Head, and Neck

Any burn of the face is dangerous since it may involve injury to the airway or the eyes. When applying gauze for burns of the face or head, avoid covering the nostrils as the victim may already be having respiratory problems. Victims with respiratory illnesses will be placed in greater jeopardy when exposed to heated air or chemical vapors. Victims with other health problems such as heart disease, kidney disease, or diabetes will react more severely to burn damage. Treat all burns as more serious if accompanied by other injuries.

To dress a burn of the face or head, proceed as follows:

- Apply several layers of gauze to the burned area and ensure that the gauze is placed between raw surfaces of ears and head.
- Loosely apply a cravat bandage around the forehead to secure layers of gauze for the upper part of the face.
- Loosely apply a second cravat bandage around the chin to secure layers of gauze for the lower part of the face.

If the neck only is burned:

- Apply gauze or other burn dressing.
- The burn dressing should be applied in several layers and covered with a cravat bandage the same as for wounds and bleeding of the neck.
- Burn dressings should always be applied loosely.

Burns to the Back

For burns to the back, apply gauze in several layers

and ensure that it covers all burned surfaces including between the arm and chest wall and in the armpit. Cover the gauze dressings with a cover dressing as follows:

- Split the apex of a triangular bandage just far enough to tie around the front of neck.
- Place the base of bandage around the lower part of the back and tie in front.
- Dress small burns of the back loosely with a triangular or cravat bandage as for wounds and bleeding between shoulders or wounds of the back as the injury may indicate.

Burns on the Chest

For burns on the chest, apply gauze in several layers and ensure that it covers all burned surfaces including between the arm and chest wall and in the armpit. Cover the gauze dressing with a cover dressing as follows:

- Split the apex of a bandage just enough to tie at the back of neck.
- Place base of bandage around the waist and tie in back.
- Dress small burns of the chest loosely with a triangular cravat bandage as for wounds and bleeding between the shoulders or wounds of the chest as the injury may indicate.

Treatment of all Other Burns

Burn dressings should be loosely covered with a bandage as described for a wound and bleeding of the part or parts involved.

Sprains, Strains, and Fractures

The musculoskeletal system is composed of all the bones, joints, muscles, tendons, ligaments, and cartilages in the body. The makeup of the musculoskeletal system is subject to injury from sprains, strains, fractures and dislocations.

Sprains

Sprains are injuries due to stretching or tearing ligaments or other tissues at a joint. They are caused by a sudden twist or stretch of a joint beyond its normal range of motion.

Sprains may be minor, causing discomfort for only a few hours. In severe cases, however, they may require many weeks of medical care.

The symptoms of a sprain are as follows:

- Pain on movement
- Swelling
- Tenderness
- Discoloration

Sprains present basically the same signs as a closed fracture. If you cannot determine whether the injury is a fracture or a sprain, treat it as a fracture.

The first aid for sprains is as follows:

- Elevate the injured area and place it at complete rest.
- Reduce swelling and relieve pain by applying an ice bag, a cloth wrung in cold water or a chemical cold pack. **Caution: Never use ice in direct contact with the skin; always wrap it in a towel or other material.**
- If swelling and pain persist, take the victim to the doctor.

286

The ankle is the part of the body most commonly affected by sprains. When the ankle has been sprained and the injured person must use the foot temporarily to reach a place for further treatment, the following care should be given:

- Unlace the shoe, but do not remove it.
- Place the center of a narrow cravat bandage under the foot in front of the heel of the shoe.
- Carry the ends up and back of the ankle, crossing above the heel, then forward, crossing over the instep, and then downward toward the arch to make a hitch under the cravat on each side, just in front of the heel of the shoe.
- Pull tightly and carry the ends back across the instep.
- Tie at the back of the ankle.

Strains

A strain is an injury to a muscle or a tendon caused by overexertion. In severe cases muscles or tendons are torn and the muscle fibers are stretched. Strains are caused by sudden movements or overexertion.

The symptoms of a strain are as follows:

- Intense pain
- Moderate swelling
- Painful and difficult movement
- Sometimes, discoloration

The first aid care for a strain is as follows:

- Place the victim in a comfortable position.
- Apply a hot, wet towel.
- Keep the injured area at rest.
- Seek medical attention.

Fractures

A fracture is a broken or cracked bone. For first aid purposes fractures can be divided into two classifications:

- Open, or compound fracture. The bone is broken and an open wound is present. Often the end of the broken bone protrudes from the wound.
- Closed, or simple fracture. No open wound is present, but there is a broken or cracked bone.

Broken bones, especially the long bones of the upper and lower extremities, often have sharp, sawtooth edges; even slight movement may cause the sharp edges to cut into blood vessels, nerves, or muscles, and perhaps through the skin. Careless or improper handling can convert a closed fracture into an open fracture, causing damage to surrounding blood vessels or nerves which can make the injury much more serious. A person handling a fracture should always keep this in mind. Damage due to careless handling of a closed fracture may greatly increase pain and shock, cause complications that will prolong the period of disability, and endanger life through hemorrhage of surrounding blood vessels.

If the broken ends of the bone extend through an open wound, there is little doubt that the victim has suffered a fracture. However, the bone does not always extend through the skin, so the person administering first aid must be able to recognize other signs that a fracture exists.

The general signs and symptoms of a fracture are as follows:

- Pain or tenderness in the region of the fracture

- Deformity or irregularity of the affected area
- Loss of function (disability) of the affected area
- Moderate or severe swelling
- Discoloration
- Information from the victim who victim may have felt the bone snap or break.

Be careful when examining injured persons, particularly those apparently suffering from fractures. For all fractures the first aider must remember to maintain an open airway, control bleeding and treat for shock. Do not attempt to change the position of an injured person until he or she has been examined and it has been determined that movement will not complicate the injuries. If the victim is lying down, it is far better to attend to the injuries with the victim in that position and with as little movement as possible. If fractures are present, make any necessary movement in such a manner as to protect the injured part against further injury.

Splints

Use splints to support, immobilize, and protect parts with injuries such as known or suspected fractures, dislocations or severe sprains. When in doubt, treat the injury as a fracture and splint it. Splints prevent movement at the area of the injury and at the nearest joints. Splints should immobilize and support the joint or bones above and below the break.

Many types of splints are available commercially. Easily applied and quickly inflated plastic splints give support to injured limbs. Improvised splints may be made from pieces of wood, broom handles, newspapers, heavy cardboard, boards, magazines, or similar firm materials.

Certain guidelines should be followed when splinting:

- Gently remove all clothing from around any suspected fracture or dislocation.
- Do not attempt to push bones back through an open wound.
- Do not attempt to straighten any fracture.
- Cover open wounds with a sterile dressing before splinting.
- Pad splints with soft material to prevent excessive pressure on the affected area and to aid in supporting the injured part.
- Pad under all natural arches of the body such as the knee and wrist.
- Support the injured part while splint is being applied.
- Splint firmly, but not so tightly as to interfere with circulation or cause undue pain.
- Support fracture or dislocation before transporting victim.
- Elevate the injured part and apply ice when possible.

Use inflatable splints to immobilize fractures of the lower leg or forearm. When applying inflatable splints (non-zipper type), follow these guidelines:

- Put splint on your own arm so that the bottom edge is above your wrist.
- Help support the victim's limb or have someone else hold it.
- Hold injured limb, and slide the splint from your forearm over the victim's injured limb.
- Inflate by mouth only to the desired pressure. The splint should be inflated to the point where

your thumb would make a slight indentation.
- Do not use an inflatable plastic splint with an open fracture with protruding bones.

For a zipper-type air splint, lay the victim's limb in the unzippered air splint, zip it and inflate. Traction cannot be maintained with this type of splint.

Change in temperature can affect air splints. Going from a cold area to a warm area will cause the splint to expand or vice versa, therefore, it may be necessary to deflate or inflate the splint until proper pressure is reached.

Areas of Fracture

Skull

A fracture may occur to any area of the skull and is considered serious due to possible injury to the brain. Injuries to the back of the head are particularly dangerous since a fractured skull may result without a visible wound to the scalp. The victim of a skull fracture may exhibit any or all of the following symptoms:

- Loss of consciousness for any length of time
- Difficulty in breathing
- Clear or blood-tinged fluid coming from the nose and/or ears
- Partial or complete paralysis
- Pupils of unequal size
- Speech disturbance
- Convulsions
- Vomiting
- Impaired vision or sudden blindness

Consider all serious injuries to the head as possible fractures of the skull. A person with a skull fracture

may also have an injury to the neck and spine.
The first aid for a skull fracture is as follows:

- Stabilize the head as you open the airway using the modified jaw-thrust maneuver.
- Check breathing - restore if necessary.
- Check pulse.
- Control bleeding from the scalp with minimal pressure and dress the wound; tie the knots of the bandage away from injured area. Do not try to control bleeding from ears or nose.
- Keep the victim quiet and lying down.
- Maintain an open airway.
- Immobilize head, neck, and back on backboard.
- Elevate the head end of the stretcher.
- Never give a stimulant.
- Keep the victim warm and treat for shock.
- Pad around the fractured area and under the neck to keep victim's head from resting on suspected fracture.

Spinal Column

The spinal column consists of bones called vertebrae. Each vertebra surrounds and protects the spinal cord and specific nerve roots.

Fracture of the spinal column may occur at any point along the backbone between its junction with the head at the top and with the pelvic basin below. Where portions of the broken vertebrae are displaced, the spinal cord may be cut, or pressure may be put on the cord.

Spinal cord injuries can result in paralysis or death, because they cannot always be corrected by surgery and the spinal cord has very limited self healing powers. Thus, it is extremely important for the person giving first aid to be able to recognize the signs of spinal column damage.

The following signs and symptoms are associated with spinal injuries:

- Pain and tenderness at the site of the injury
- Deformity
- Cuts and bruises
- Paralysis

First, check the lower extremities for paralysis. If the victim is conscious, use the following method:

- Ask the victim if he or she can feel your touch on his or her feet.
- Ask the victim to wiggle his or her toes.
- Ask the victim to press against your hand with his or her feet.

Second, check the upper extremities for paralysis. If the victim is conscious, use the following method:

- Ask the victim if he or she can feel your touch to his or her hands.
- Ask the victim to wiggle his or her fingers.
- Ask the victim to grasp your hand and squeeze.

If the victim is unconscious, perform the following tests for paralysis:

- Stroke the soles of the feet or ankles with a pointed object; if the spinal cord is undamaged, the feet will react.
- Stroke the palms of the hands with a pointed object; if the spinal cord is undamaged, the hands will react.

Treat all questionable injuries to the spinal column, even in the absence of signs of paralysis, as a fracture of the spinal column. The initial care that the victim receives at the scene of the accident is extremely important. Proper care, not speed, is essential. Improper care or handling could result in paralysis or death. The first aid for an individual with a fractured spinal column uses fifteen bandages as follows:

- If a broken-back splint is used, pad each long board with a blanket.
- Stabilize the head, immobilizing it in line with the rest of the body. Maintain stabilization until after the victim is secured to a splint, stretcher, or other hard, flat surface which provides firm support. Do not move victim until completely immobilized.
- Use a blanket or padding around the head and neck. Fold to make a strip about six inches wide and long enough to run along the side of the head from the shoulder to the head, across the top of the head and down the other side to the shoulder.

immobilize head
(rolled blanket or pad)

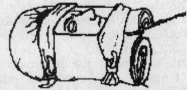

- Pass first bandage around the forehead padding and splint, and tie on the outer side of splint.
- Pass second bandage around the splint and padding at the chin, and tie on the outer side of splint.

- Pass third bandage around the body and well up in the armpits and tie on outer side of splint.
- Pass fourth bandage around the body and splint at the lower part of the chest and tie on the outer side of the splint.
- Pass the fifth bandage around the body and splint at the hips, and tie on the outer side of the splint.
- Pass the center of the sixth bandage well up on the shoulder, passing one end between the long boards under the neck, continuing under the crosspiece, completing the tie at the upper edge of splint under the armpit.
- Tie the seventh bandage in the same manner around the other shoulder.
- Pass the eighth bandage around one hip and crotch and crosspiece between long boards and tie on outer side of splint.
- Apply ninth bandage in the same manner around the other hip.
- Apply tenth bandage around the upper part of one thigh and the long board and tie on the outer side of the splint.
- Apply eleventh bandage on the other side in the same manner.
- Pass twelfth bandage around the leg and long board just below the knee and tie on the outer side of the splint.
- Apply thirteenth bandage on the other side in the same manner.
- Pass the fourteenth bandage around one ankle and the long board, and tie on the outer side of the splint.

- Apply fifteenth bandage on the other side in the same manner.
- Use enough people to safely lift the victim as a unit and place the victim on his or her back on the splint or stretcher.
- Lift victim only high enough to slide the splint or stretcher underneath.
- Secure the victim to the splint or stretcher so that the entire body is immobilized.
- Cover with a blanket and treat for shock.

Nose

A broken nose is a very common type of fracture and may result from any hard blow. The symptoms of a broken nose are as follows:

- Deformity of the bridge of the nose
- Pain
- Bleeding
- Swelling

Treat any blow to the nose that causes bleeding as a fracture.

The first aid care for a broken nose is as follows:

- Apply a bandage compress if there is an open fracture.
- Take the victim to the doctor.

Upper Jaw

In fractures of the upper jaw or cheekbone, where there is an open wound, treat as for an open wound of the face, but do not tie bandage knots over wounds. If there is no open wound, a dressing is not necessary, but take the victim to a doctor.

Lower Jaw

The symptoms of a fracture of the lower jaw are as

follows:
- The mouth is usually open.
- Saliva mixed with blood flows from the mouth.
- The teeth of the lower jaw may be uneven, loosened, or knocked out.
- Talking is painful and difficult.

The first aid for a fracture of the lower jaw is as follows:
- Maintain a clear airway.
- Gently place the jaw in a position so that the lower teeth rest against the upper teeth, if possible.
- Place the center of a cravat bandage over the front of the chin and pass the ends around the back of the head and tie, leaving the ends long.
- Place the center of a second cravat bandage under the chin, pass the ends over the cheeks to the center of the top of the head and tie, leaving the ends long.
- Bring the ends of the two bandages together and tie separately. Do not tie too tightly.
- Transport the victim on his or her side to allow drainage if no spinal injury is suspected.

Collarbone

Fracture of the collarbone frequently is caused by a fall with the hand outstretched or by a blow to the shoulder. The symptoms of a fractured collarbone are as follows:
- Pain in the area of the shoulder
- Partial or total disability of the arm on the injured side
- The injured shoulder tends to droop forward.
- The victim frequently supports the arm on the

injured side at the elbow or wrist with the other hand.

Support the fracture until the following dressings have been applied:

- Place padding between the arm and the victim's side.
- Put the arm on the injured side in a triangular sling with the hand elevated about four to five inches.

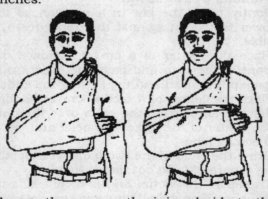

- Secure the arm on the injured side to the body with a medium cravat. Center the bandage on the outside of the arm. Carry the bandage across the chest and back. Tie over a pad on the uninjured side of the body.

Shoulder Blade

Fracture of the shoulder blade is not a common injury. It is sometimes caused by a direct blow to the shoulder blade and usually results in a closed fracture with little displacement. Symptoms are as follows:

- Pain and swelling at the fracture
- Inability to swing the arm back and forth from the shoulder

To support a fracture of the shoulder blade proceed as follows:

- Place the forearm in a triangular sling.

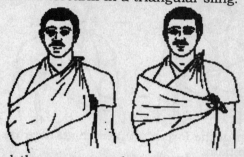

- Bind the arm securely to the chest with a wide cravat bandage extending from the point of the shoulder downward by carrying one end across the chest and the other end across the back.
- Tie over a pad under the opposite armpit.

Upper Arm

Fracture of the upper portion of the arm is recognized by the following symptoms:

- Swelling
- Deformity
- Inability to use the arm below the point of the fracture.

In order to immobilize a fracture of the upper third of the arm proceed as follows:

- Have an assistant support the fracture on both sides of the break.

- Bind the arm to the rib cage with a wide cravat bandage that is tied over a pad under the opposite armpit.
- Place the forearm in a cravat bandage sling.

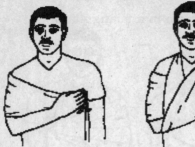 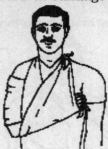

Do not pull the forearm up too high because this will increase pain.

Lower Arm, Elbow, Forearm, or Wrist

Take extreme care when dealing with a fractured elbow, as the fracture may cause extensive damage to surrounding tissues, nerves, and blood vessels. Improper care and handling of a fractured elbow could result in a permanent disability.

The symptoms of a fractured elbow are as follows:

- Extreme pain
- Extensive discoloration around elbow
- Swelling
- Deformity
- Bone may be visible or project from the wound.

The first aid for a fractured elbow in a straight position is as follows:

- Do not bend, straighten, or twist the arm in any direction.

- If available, apply an inflatable plastic splint.
- If an inflatable plastic splint is not available, use a splint long enough to reach from one inch below the armpit to one inch beyond the tip of the middle finger.
- While the fracture is being supported, pad to conform to the deformity and place splint on the inner side of the arm.
- Place the center of the first cravat bandage on the outside of the arm at the upper end of the splint, cross on the inside of the arm over the splint, pass the ends one or more times around the arm and splint, and tie on the outside.
- Place the centers of the second and third cravat bandages on the arm just above and below the elbow, and apply in a similar manner.
- Center the fourth cravat bandage on the back of the wrist. Pass the ends around and cross on the splint under the wrist, bring one end up around the little finger side, and cross over the back of the hand and down between the forefinger and thumb. Pass the other end up over the thumb, cross it over the back of the hand down around the little finger side, then cross both ends on the splint and tie on top of the hand.
- Tie a fifth cravat bandage around the splint, arm and body to prevent movement during transportation.

If the arm is bent, immobilize in a bent position by making an L-shaped splint for the forearm and wrist from two pieces of board one-half inch thick and four inches wide. One piece should be long enough to extend from one inch below the armpit to the point of the elbow and the other long enough to extend from the point of the elbow to one inch beyond the end of the middle finger. Immobilize the limb to the splint in the following manner:

- Fasten the boards together securely to form an L-shaped splint.
- Pad the splint.
- While an assistant supports the fracture on both sides of the break apply the splint to the inner side of the arm and forearm after placing the forearm across the chest.
- Use four cravat bandages to hold the splint in place.
- Place the center of the first cravat bandage on the outside of the arm at the upper end of the splint, pass around the arm one or more times, and tie on the arm.
- Place the centers of the second and third cravat bandages on the arm and forearm, respectively, passing around one or more times and tying on the arm.
- Apply the fourth cravat bandage by placing the center of the bandage on the back of the wrist, passing the ends around and crossing on the splint under the wrist. Take one end up around the little finger side, passing over the back of the hand and down between the forefinger and thumb. Pass the other end up over the thumb, and cross it over the back of the hand down around the little finger side; then cross both ends on the splint and tie on top of the hand.
- Place the arm in a cravat bandage sling.

Fractures of the forearm and wrist are usually less

painful than fractures of the arm, shoulder blade, or elbow. The symptoms of a fractured forearm and wrist are as follows:

- Pain
- Tenderness
- Severe deformity, especially if both bones of the forearm are broken

If available, use a plastic inflatable splint to immobilize the forearm or wrist.

Hand and Fingers

Fractures of the hand usually result from a direct blow. The symptoms of a fracture of the hand are as follows:

- Acute pain
- Tenderness
- Swelling
- Discoloration
- Enlarged joints

If available, use a plastic inflatable splint for immobilization.

Use a board splint if a plastic inflatable splint is not available. To immobilize a fractured hand with a board splint, proceed as follows:

- Apply a well-padded splint about one-half inch thick, four inches wide, and long enough to reach from the point of the elbow to one inch beyond the end of the middle finger.
- Place padding in the palm of the hand and under the wrist.
- Carry one end around the little finger side across the back of the hand and wrist and the other end around the thumb side across the back of the hand and wrist.

- Cross the ends on the inside of the wrist, bring them to the back of the wrist and tie.
- Bring the apex down over the knot and tuck it under.
- Place the forearm in a cravat bandage sling.
- Apply the splint to the inside of the forearm and hand with one cravat and one triangular bandage.
- Place the center of the cravat on the outside of the forearm just below the elbow; pass it around the forearm one or more times; tie it on the outside of the forearm.
- Place the base of a triangular bandage under the splint at the wrist; bring the apex around the end of the splint over the hand to a point above the wrist.
- Carry one end around the little finger side across the back of the hand and wrist and the other end around the thumb side across the back of the hand and wrist.
- Cross the ends on the inside of the wrist, bring them to the back of the wrist and tie.
- Bring the apex down over the knot and tuck it under.
- Place the forearm in a cravat bandage sling.

Finger

The symptoms of a fracture of the finger is as follows:

- Pain
- Swelling
- Deformity

The first aid for a fractured finger is as follows:

- Place a narrow padded splint under the broken

finger and palm of the hand.
- Pass a narrow strip of cloth around the splint and palm of the hand; tie over the splint.
- Pass a narrow strip of cloth around the finger and the splint above the fracture; tie over the splint.
- Pass a narrow strip of cloth around the finger and the splint below the fracture; tie over the splint.
- Place the hand in a narrow cravat bandage sling.

Rib

Fracture of a rib usually is caused by a direct blow or a severe squeeze. A fracture can occur at any point along the rib. The symptoms of a fractured rib are as follows:
- Severe pain on breathing
- Tenderness over the fracture
- Deformity
- Inability to take a deep breath

Cravat bandages will immobilize fractured ribs. Place the bandages in the following order:
- Apply padding over injured ribs.
- Apply two medium cravat bandages around the chest firmly enough to afford support, centering the cravats on either side of the pain.
- Upon exhalation, tie the knots over a pad on the opposite side of the body. If the cravat bandages cause more pain, loosen them.
- Support the arm on the injured side in a sling.
- Treat for shock as it is usually severe.
- Secure medical treatment.

Wrap the chest gently when the ribs are depressed or frothy blood comes from the victim's mouth. These may be indications of a punctured lung. Place the victim in a semi-prone position (if no neck or spine injury exists) with the injured side down. This will allow more room for expansion of the uninjured lung.

Pelvis or Hip

Fracture of the pelvis or hip usually results from a squeezing type injury through the hips or from a direct blow. Use extreme care when handling an individual with a fracture of the pelvis or hip because there is a possibility of associated internal injuries to the digestive, urinary, or genital organs. The symptoms of a fractured pelvis or hip are as follows:

- Pain in the pelvic region
- Discoloration
- Unable to raise his or her leg
- Inward rotation of foot and leg on affected side

To support the pelvic region before the victim is transported proceed as follows:

- Maintain support of the pelvic region with hands at the sides of the hips until two wide bandages have been applied.
- Place the center of a wide cravat bandage over one hip, the upper edge extending about two inches above the crest of the hip bone.
- Pass the ends around the body and tie over a pad on the opposite hip.
- Place the center of a second wide cravat bandage over the opposite hip, the upper edge extending about two inches above the crest of the hipbone.

- Pass the ends around the body and tie on the first bandage.
- Lift the victim only high enough to place him or her on a firm support, preferably a broken back splint.
- When a broken back splint is used, secure the body to the splint with eight cravat bandages as follows:
- Pass the first cravat bandage around the splint and the upper part of the chest, well up in the armpits and tie on one side near the splint.
- Pass the second cravat bandage around the splint and the lower part of the chest and tie near the splint.
- Pass the third and fourth cravat bandages around the splint and each thigh just below the crotch and tie on the outside near the splint.
- Pass the fifth and sixth cravat bandages around splint and each leg, just below the knee and tie on the outside near the splint.
- Pass the seventh and eighth cravat bandages around the splint and each ankle, and tie on the outside near the splint.
- Cover the victim with a blanket and treat for shock.
- Get the victim to the doctor or hospital.

Thigh or Knee

If a fracture of the thigh or knee is open, dress the wound. If the fracture is at the knee joint and the limb is not in a straight position, make no attempt to straighten the limb. Splint in line of deformity. Attempts to straighten the limb may increase the possibility of permanent damage. Improvise a way to immobilize the knee as it is found, using padding to fill any space. Use the utility splint stretcher or a similar support to immobilize fractures of the knee or thigh. Before placing the victim on the stretcher, it should be well padded and tested. Additional padding will also be necessary for the natural arches of the body. Raise the victim carefully for placement on the stretcher while the fracture is supported from the underside on both sides of the break.

Apply the splint with bandages. All bandages should be tied on the injured side near the splint.

- Tie the first bandage around the body and splint under the armpits.
- Tie the second around the chest and splint and the third around the hips and splint.
- Tie the fourth and fifth bandages on the injured leg just below the crotch at the thigh and above the knee, respectively, (above and below fracture) and tie on the injured side near the splint.
- Tie the sixth and seventh bandages on the injured leg below the knee and at the ankle.
- An additional bandage at the ankle on the uninjured side may be needed for additional support.
- The victim should be transported on a regular stretcher or stretcher board.

When using a stretcher board, it should be well padded and the bandages applied in normal order. On some types of stretcher boards it may be necessary to tie both lower limbs together with each of the last four cravat bandages. To prevent movement of the legs, pad well between the legs before applying the cravats.

Any improvised splint for the thigh or knee should be long enough to immobilize the hip and the ankle.

Kneecap

A splint suitable for a broken back may also be used for a fracture of the kneecap. Dress any open wound first. The splint should be well padded with additional padding under all natural body arches. Support the fracture from the top and on both sides and carefully raise the victim to place the prepared and tested splint underneath.

Apply the splint with seven cravat bandages. Tie all bandages on the injured side near the splint, except the fifth and sixth bandages which tie on top.

- Tie three bandages around the body and the splint; one just below the armpits, one around the chest, and one around the hips.
- Tie the fourth bandage around the thigh and splint just below the crotch.
- Place the center of the fifth bandage just above the kneecap, bring the ends under the thigh and splint, and bring ends over the leg above the kneecap, but do not tie.
- Place the center of the sixth bandage just below the kneecap, bring the ends under the leg and splint up over the thigh and tie above the knee over the fifth bandage.
- Pull the ends of the fifth bandage tight and tie below the knee over the sixth bandage.
- The seventh bandage is tied around the ankle and splint.
- An additional bandage at the ankle and thigh on the uninjured side may be needed for additional support.

Transport the victim on a regular stretcher. Any stretcher board used for this type of injury should be the type of board which is prepared for individual bandaging of each lower extremity. Otherwise, the bandages would be applied as for fracture of thigh or knee. Any improvised splint for the kneecap should be long enough to immobilize the hip and the ankle.

Leg or Ankle

If the fracture is open, dress the wound before splinting. When it is necessary to remove a shoe or boot because of pain from swelling of the ankle or for any other reason, the removal must be carefully done by unlacing or cutting the boot to prevent damage to the ankle. In the absence of severe swelling or bleeding it may be wise to leave the boot on for additional support.

The splint for a fracture of the leg or ankle should reach from against the buttocks to beyond the heel. Place a well-padded splint under the victim while the leg is supported on both sides of the fracture. Tie the bandages on the outer side, near the splint as follows:

- Pass the end of the first bandage around the inner side of the thigh at the groin, pass it over the thigh under the splint, and tie.
- Pass two bandages around the thigh and splint, one at the middle of the thigh and the other just above the knee and tie.
- Place additional padding around the knee and ankle.
- Place a padded splint on the outer side of the leg.
- Pass a fourth bandage around the leg, the pad-

ding, and the splint just below the knee and tie; pass a fifth bandage just above or below the fracture and tie. **Do not** tie over fracture.

- Pass the center of a sixth bandage around the instep and bring the ends up each side of the ankle.
- Cross the ends on top and pass them around the ankle and splint.
- Cross the ends under the splint, return to the top of the ankle, cross and carry down each side of the ankle and tie under the instep.

When using an inflatable plastic splint, roll up or cut away the clothing from the limb to a point above the upper end of the splint. The splint should be long enough to immobilize the knee as well as the ankle. Cover open wounds with gauze, but they need not be bandaged because the splint will form an airtight cover for such wounds. After the splint is applied, pressure from the inflated splint will help control any bleeding that may develop. Apply the splint while supporting the fracture on both sides. Close and inflate the splint.

Ankle or Foot

To make an improvised splint for the ankle or foot, proceed as follows:

- Carefully fold a blanket or pillow around the ankle and foot.
- Tie the first bandage around the leg above the ankle.
- Tie the second bandage around the ankle.
- Tie the third bandage below the ankle.
- Place padding between the ankles and extend the padding above the knees.

- Place the fourth bandage around knees and tie.
- Place the fifth bandage below knees and tie.
- Place the sixth bandage around ankles and tie.

Dislocations

A dislocation is when one or more of the bones forming a joint slip out of normal position. The ligaments holding the bones in proper position are stretched and sometimes torn loose. Fractures are often associated with dislocations.

Dislocations may result from the following:

- Force applied at or near the joint
- Sudden muscular contractions
- Twisting strains on joint ligaments
- Falls where the force of landing is transferred to a joint

Some general symptoms of dislocations are as follows:

- Rigidity and loss of function
- Deformity
- Pain
- Swelling
- Tenderness
- Discoloration

General First Aid for Dislocations

A first aider does not have the skill necessary to reduce dislocations. Inexperience in manipulating the joints can further damage the ligaments, blood vessels and nerves found close to joints. With one exception (the lower jaw) only a physician should reduce a dislocation. The victim experiences pain which justifies one reduction attempt.

Splint and/or dress the affected joint in line of deformity in which you find it. Obtain medical help.

Lower Jaw

The symptoms of a dislocated lower jaw are as follows:

- Pain
- Open mouth
- Rigid jaw
- Difficulty in speaking

If medical aid is not available for some time, reduce the dislocation as follows:

- Place thumbs in the victim's mouth, resting them well back on each side of the lower teeth.
- Seize the outside of the lower jaw with the fingers. Press first downward and forward.
- When the jaw starts into place, slip the thumbs off the teeth to the inside of the cheeks.
- Remove thumbs from mouth.
- Place the center of a cravat bandage over the front of the chin.
- Carry the ends to the back of the head and tie.
- Center another bandage under the victim's chin, bring the ends to the top of the head and tie.
- Bring the ends of both bandages together and tie them separately.

NOTE: If the reduction attempt is not successful, do not make repeated attempts to reduce the dislocation and do not apply a dressing. Secure medical treatment.

Shoulder

The shoulder joint usually is dislocated by falls or blows directly on the shoulder or by falls on the hand or elbow. The symptoms of a dislocated shoulder are as follows:

- The elbow stands off one or two inches from the body.
- The arm is held rigid.
- The shoulder appears flat.
- A marked depression is evident beneath the point of the shoulder.
- Pain and swelling are present at the site of the injury.
- The victim cannot bring the elbow in contact with the side.

While the arm is being supported in the position in which it was found, immobilize the shoulder in the following manner:

- Place the point of a wedge-shaped pad (approximately four inches wide and one to three inches thick) between the arm and the body.
- Tape or tie the pad in place.
- Place the center of a medium width cravat on the outside of the arm just above the elbow.
- Carry one end across the chest and the other end across the back.
- Tie on the opposite side over a pad.
- Place the arm in a triangular bandage sling.

Elbow

Dislocation occurs at the elbow joint as a result of a blow at the joint or occasionally by a fall on the hand. It usually can be recognized by these symptoms:

- Deformity at the joint
- Inability to bend the limb at the joint
- Great pain

The elbow must be immobilized in the line the deformity is found. While the elbow is being supported, proceed as follows:

- Prepare and pad a splint, straight, L-shaped, or a modification of the latter depending on the position of the arm, long enough to reach from one inch below the armpit to one inch beyond the tip of the middle finger.
- Pad splint to conform to the deformity, and place on the inside of the arm.
- Place the center of the first cravat bandage on the outside of the arm at the upper end of the splint, cross on the inside of the arm over the splint, pass the ends one or more times around the arm and splint, and tie on the outside.
- Place the center of the second cravat bandage on the arm just above the elbow and apply in a similar manner.
- Place the center of the third cravat bandage on the forearm just below the elbow, and apply in a similar manner.
- Place the center of the fourth cravat bandage on the back of the wrist, passing the ends around and crossing on the splint under the wrist, bring one end up around the little finger side, and cross over the back of the hand and down between the forefinger and thumb. Pass the other end up over the thumb, cross it over the back of the hand down around the little finger side, then cross both ends on the splint and tie on the top of the hand.
- Bind the limb to the body or place the forearm in a cravat bandage sling (depending on the position of the arm).

Wrist

Dislocation of the wrist usually occurs when the hand is extended to break the force of a fall. It is difficult, however, to distinguish between a dislocation and a fractured wrist. Treat a suspected dislocated wrist the same as a fractured wrist.

Finger

The usual symptoms of a dislocated finger are as follows:
- Inability to bend at dislocation
- Deformity of the joint
- Shortening of the digit
- Pain and swelling

Do not attempt to reduce the dislocation. immobilize the digit by using small pads as for any deformity and splinting, or by tying the injured member to the one next to it. Obtain medical treatment.

Hip

Dislocation of the hip usually results from falling onto the foot or knee. While supporting the dislocation in the line of deformity, carefully raise the victim only high enough to be placed on a well-padded and tested splint or stretcher board suitable for a broken back. Support is necessary until the splint or stretcher board is applied.

The symptoms of a dislocated hip are as follows:
- Intense pain
- Lengthening or shortening of the leg, with the foot turned in or out

Pain and swelling at the joint The first aid for a dislocated hip is:
- Make a pad of clothing, blankets, or other mate-

rial large enough to support the limb in the line of deformity. (The affected leg will be turned either inward or outward.)

- Place a small pad between the feet.
- Pass the first cravat bandage around the splint, the upper part of the chest, and tie the ends of the bandage on the injured side near the splint.
- Pass the second cravat bandage around the splint and lower part of the chest and tie the ends of the bandage on the injured side near the splint.
- Pass the third cravat bandage around the splint and the body at the hips, and tie on the injured side near the splint.
- Pass the fourth cravat bandage around the splint and the thigh just above the knee, and tie on the injured side near the splint.
- Pass the fifth cravat bandage around the splint and the ankles, and tie on the injured side near the splint.
- Pass the sixth cravat bandage over the insteps, cross the ends under the soles of the feet, and bring them back to the insteps, tying loosely.
- If the victim is unconscious, the forearms should be placed in a basket sling.

Knee

Dislocation of the knee results from direct force applied at the knee or from a fall on the knee. The symptoms of the dislocation are as follows:

- Deformity
- Inability to use the knee
- Great pain

While supporting the dislocation, apply a splint as

for fracture of the thigh, using either a broken back splint or a stretcher board. Place extra padding of blankets, clothes, or similar material to conform to the deformity.

Ankle

Dislocation of the ankle may show several types of deformity. Bones are almost always broken. There is a marked deformity at the joint. As a rule, there is rapid and marked swelling and great pain. While supporting the dislocation, apply an improvised splint as for a fracture of the ankle or foot, and add padding to conform to the deformity. Use an air splint long enough to immobilize the knee or use a blanket or pillow to splint the leg or ankle. Use additional cravats for anchoring to broken back splint.

Toe

The symptoms of a dislocated toe are as follows:
- Inability to bend at dislocation
- Deformity of the joint
- Shortening of the digit
- Pain and swelling

Do not attempt to reduce the dislocation. Immobilize the digit by using small pads as for any deformity and splinting it by tying the injured member to the one next to it.